Ophthalmic Radiation Therapy

Developments in Ophthalmology

Vol. 52

Series Editor

F. Bandello Milan

Ophthalmic Radiation Therapy

Techniques and Applications

Volume Editors

Arun D. Singh Cleveland, Ohio
David E. Pelayes Buenos Aires
Stefan Seregard Stockholm
Roger Macklis Cleveland, Ohio

49 figures, 42 in color, and 7 tables, 2013

KARGER

Basel · Freiburg · Paris · London · New York · New Delhi · Bangkok · Beijing · Tokyo · Kuala Lumpur · Singapore · Sydney

Arun D. Singh
Department of Ophthalmic Oncology
Cole Eye Institute
Cleveland Clinic Foundation
9500 Euclid Avenue
Cleveland, OH 44195 (USA)

David E. Pelayes
Maimonides University
Buenos Aires University
Ciudad Autonoma de Buenos Aires
Buenos Aires (Argentina)

Stefan Seregard
St Eriks Eye Hospital
Karolinska Institutet
Polhemsgatan 50
SE-11 282 Stockholm (Sweden)

Roger Macklis
Department of Ophthalmic Oncology
Cole Eye Institute
Cleveland Clinic Foundation
9500 Euclid Avenue
Cleveland, OH 44195 (USA)

Library of Congress Cataloging-in-Publication Data

Ophthalmic radiation therapy : techniques and applications / volume editors, Arun D. Singh, David E. Pelayes, Stefan Seregard, Roger Macklis.
p. ; cm. -- (Developments in ophthalmology, ISSN 0250-3751 ; vol. 52)
Includes bibliographical references and indexes.
ISBN 978-3-318-02440-1 (hard cover : alk. paper) -- ISBN 978-3-318-02441-8 (electronic version)
I. Singh, Arun D., editor of compilation. II. Pelayes, David E., editor of compilation. III. Seregard, Stefan, editor of compilation. IV. Macklis, Roger M., editor of compilation. V. Series: Developments in ophthalmology ; v. 52. 0250-3751
[DNLM: 1. Eye Neoplasms--radiotherapy. 2. Radiotherapy--methods. W1 DE998NG v.52 2013 / WW 149]
RC280.E9
616.99'484--dc23

2013024151

Bibliographic Indices. This publication is listed in bibliographic services, including Current Contents® and Index Medicus.

www.karger.com
Printed in Germany on acid-free paper by Kraft Druck GmbH, Ettlingen
ISSN 0250–3751
e-ISSN 1662–2790
ISBN 978–3–318–02440–1
e-ISBN 978–3–318–02441–8

To my parents who educated me beyond their means, my wife Annapurna,
and my children, Nakul and Rahul, who make all my efforts worthwhile. (A.D.S.)

To Veronica, love you forever. We will meet again. (D.E.P.)

To Marie, Louise and Caroline for all your love and support. (S.S.)

For our patients and our students who continue
to help us to see with clearer eyes. (R.M.)

Contents

List of Contributors

Mary E. Aronow
Department of Ophthalmic Oncology
Cole Eye Institute
Cleveland Clinic Foundation
9500 Euclid Avenue
Cleveland, OH 44195 (USA)
E-Mail turellm2@gmail.com

Ehsan H. Balagamwala
Department of Radiation Oncology
Taussig Cancer Institute
Cleveland, OH 44195 (USA)
E-Mail ehsanhb@gmail.com

Justis P. Ehlers
Vitreoretinal Service
Cleveland Clinic Cole Eye Institute
9500 Euclid Avenue
Cleveland, OH 44195 (USA)
E-Mail ehlersj@ccf.org

David Y. Kim
Retina Service
Department of Ophthalmology
Massachusetts Eye and Ear Infirmary
Harvard Medical School
Boston, MA 02114 (USA)
E-Mail David_Kim@meei.harvard.edu

Shannon M. MacDonald
Department of Radiation Oncology
Massachusetts General Hospital
Harvard Medical School
Boston, MA 02114 (USA)
E-Mail smacdonald@partners.org

Roger Macklis
Department of Ophthalmic Oncology
Cole Eye Institute
Cleveland Clinic Foundation
9500 Euclid Avenue
Cleveland, OH 44195 (USA)
E-Mail macklir@ccf.org

Gaurav Marwaha
Department of Radiation Oncology
Taussig Cancer Institute
Cleveland, OH 44195 (USA)
E-Mail marwahg2@ccf.org

Carlos A. Medina Mendez
Vitreoretinal Service
Cleveland Clinic Cole Eye Institute
9500 Euclid Avenue
Cleveland, OH 44195 (USA)
E-Mail medina25@hotmail.com

Shizuo Mukai
Retina Service
Department of Ophthalmology
Massachusetts Eye and Ear Infirmary
Harvard Medical School
Boston, MA 02114 (USA)
E-Mail Shizuo_Mukai@meei.harvard.edu

David E. Pelayes
Maimonides University
Buenos Aires University
Ciudad Autonoma de Buenos Aires
Emilio Mitre 477 5 A Caballito
Buenos Aires (Argentina)
E-Mail davidpelayes@gmail.com

Stefan Seregard
St Eriks Eye Hospital
Karolinska Institutet
Polhemsgatan 50
SE-11 282 Stockholm (Sweden)
E-Mail stefan.seregard@sankterik.se

Roshan V. Sethi
Department of Radiation Oncology
Massachusetts General Hospital
Harvard Medical School
Boston, MA 02114 (USA)
E-Mail rsethi2@partners.org

Arun D. Singh
Department of Ophthalmic Oncology
Cole Eye Institute
Cleveland Clinic Foundation
9500 Euclid Avenue
Cleveland, OH 44195 (USA)
E-Mail singha@ccf.org

Abigail Stockham
Department of Radiation Oncology
Taussig Cancer Institute
Cleveland, OH 44195 (USA)
E-Mail stockha@ccf.org

Allan Wilkinson
Department of Radiation Oncology
Taussig Cancer Institute
Cleveland, OH 44195 (USA)
E-Mail wilkina@ccf.org

Foreword

The physicist W.C. Roentgen discovered X-rays in 1895, which were first named after him mainly in the German-speaking literature. The idea of using X-rays in the treatment of malignant diseases was born in the same year when, upon the initiative of a medical student in Chicago named Emil Grubber, X-rays were used to treat a local relapse of breast cancer. Already in 1897, H. Chalupecki published his experimental results about the effect of the new radiation treatment on rabbit eyes. H.L. Hilgartner wrote the first clinical report on the treatment of a bilateral retinoblastoma with X-rays in 1903. At first, there was a general uncertainty about the exact dosage needed so that medical application only slowly gained general acceptance. The introduction of a unit to calculate the absorbed energy within the irradiated tissue – today measured in 'Grays' (1 Gy = 1 Ws/kg) – has been a great step forward.

Furthermore, we had to learn that the biological radiation effect is not only dependent on the absorbed energy, but also on the quality of the rays (ionization density, LET), the dose distribution in time (protraction, fractionation), extension of the radiation field as well as some other factors. For this reason, the term relative biological effectiveness was created. The introduction of brachytherapy with radium contact treatment by Mme S. Laborde in Villejuif in 1925, X-ray brachytherapy by H. Chaoul in 1935, and finally the development of the precise irradiation technique for eyelid cancer by F. Baclesse of the Foundation Curie in Paris in 1939 brought forward the supposition to considerably improve the results after radiation treatment in patients suffering from cancer of the eyelid.

In 1958, A.B. Reese from New York recommended specially shaped irradiation tubes and, with the so-called cross fire technique, was able to considerably improve the outcome after X-ray treatment of children suffering from retinoblastoma. In 1983, J. Schipper was the first to introduce precision megavoltage external beam radiation therapy for retinoblastoma.

The use of radon seeds by R.F. Moore, H.B. Stallard and J.G. Milner in 1931 provided a new method for the treatment of intraocular melanomas using brachytherapy and thus avoiding enucleation. In 1960, H.B. Stallard presented his first patients suffering from choroidal melanoma who had been treated successfully by shell-shaped ^{60}Co applicators sutured onto the scleral surface at the base of the intraocular tumor.

The ball-shaped ^{60}Co applicators developed by B. Rosengreen and B. Tengroth did not gain acceptance. Unfortunately, these gamma ray sources caused severe radiation-induced side effects in the course of time. For this reason, a number of alternative radionuclides were introduced to improve therapeutic outcome: ^{106}Ru/^{106}Rh plaques by P.K. Lommatzsch, R. Vollmar and G. Vormum, ^{125}I plaques by M. Rothman and S. Packer, ^{192}Ir plaques by D. Grange, ^{90}Sr/^{90}Y plaques by L. Missotten, ^{103}Pa plaques by P. Finger, and finally the binuclid applicator (^{106}Ru/^{106}Rh in combination with ^{125}I) by N. Bornfeld. Herewith, the functional results could be remarkably improved, especially in cases with small and medium-sized tumors. H.L. Friedell, C.J. Thomas and J.S. Krohmer constructed some concave mirror-like ^{90}Sr/90Y applicators. With them, M. Lederman from the Royal Marsden Hospital in London considerably improved his postradiation results in eyes with conjunctival melanomas, as reported 1966.

C. Haye, H. Jammet and M.A. Dollfus published their two volumes of 'L'oil et les radiations ionisantes' in 1965 and lay the theoretical and practical foundations for radiation therapy of malignant eye tumors.

The introduction of particulate radiation into medicine was an important step forward. Taking advantage of the 'Bragg peak', we were enabled to optimize the dose distribution even within larger intraocular tumors, and at the same to protect structures of the eye from not being involved in the malignant tumor. E.S. Gragoudas introduced proton beam therapy in 1978 and D.H. Char the use of accelerated helium ions in 1986 for the treatment of intraocular melanomas. In addition, the development of stereotactic radiation techniques either with the linear accelerator (LINAC) or with the gamma knife (^{60}Co) gave us the opportunity to optimize the tumor dose in a similar fashion as the much more expensive proton beams.

Radiotherapy of choroidal melanomas can destroy the local tumor; however, it does not prevent the patients from death due to metastasis in about 50% (Collaborative Ocular Melanoma Study Group, 2004). Monosomy in chromosome 3 and gain of chromosome 8 in melanoma cells are significant features when seeking an increased probability for the development of metastases, as we have recently seen in the results of numerous publications, especially those by B. Horsthemke, E. Passarge and N. Bornfeld. Consequently, human genetic examinations of tissue from choroidal melanomas become increasingly important to detect micro metastases, thus enabling to commence an effective adjuvant treatment in patients with a high risk of developing metastases.

The management of patients with an ophthalmic tumor can be particularly challenging. That is why intensive cooperation between experienced ophthalmologists, radiologists and radiation physicists is a necessary and fundamental condition to successfully utilize all types of ionizing radiation in order to treat tumors of the eye and its adnexa. Because of the slow regression of most tumors after irradiation as well as the chance of tumor recurrence and radiation-induced side effects, it seems mandatory to perform well-organized follow-up examinations of each irradiated patient.

The last comprehensive book on this topic, *'Radiotherapy of Intraocular and Orbital Tumors'*, was published by E. Alberti and R.H. Sagerman in 1993. Since then, 20 years have passed and many new therapeutic procedures and a lot of clinical trials have appeared in the literature.

Therefore, we welcome Arun D. Singh as an international experienced colleague who is well noted in the field of ophthalmic oncology for taking the initiative to compose and present our current knowledge of radiation therapy in ophthalmology in this volume of *Developments in Ophthalmology*.

He has made use of his good reputation to bring together eminent experts from around the world to produce an up-to-date and comprehensive overview of radiation therapy in ophthalmology.

This book will be most valuable not only to trainees but also to mature ophthalmologists, oncologists, radiologists and other specialists participating in the care of patients, especially those with ophthalmic tumors.

Only a well-founded knowledge of all the pros and cons of ionizing radiation for medical purposes can meet the requirements to apply radiotherapy properly.

In any case, the principle in medicine 'nihil nocere' should be especially noted.

Peter K. Lommatzsch, MD, Leipzig

Preface

Ophthalmic tumors are rare and diverse, hence their diagnosis and treatment usually requires special expertise and equipment, and in many instances is controversial. Increasingly, the care of such patients is provided by a multidisciplinary team, comprising ocular oncologists, general oncologists, radiation therapists, radiation oncologists and other specialists. The field of radiation oncology is advancing rapidly, because of accelerating progress in tumor biology, pharmacology, and instrumentation. For all these reasons, we felt that there was scope for a monograph dedicated to radiation therapy of ocular tumors, offering a comprehensive source of authoritative information on the subject of ocular and adnexal radiation therapy.

This monograph, a conjoint effort of ocular oncologists and radiation oncologists, comprises of 10 chapters covering basic and advanced radiation therapy techniques followed by specific indications by location (uveal, retinal, orbital tumors, eyelid and conjunctival tumors) and complications of radiation therapy. We have also included a chapter on investigational use of radiation therapy for age-related macular degeneration.

It is our sincere hope that readers will find as much pleasure reading this textbook as we had writing and editing it.

Arun D. Singh, MD, Cleveland, Ohio, USA
David E. Pelayes, MD, PhD, Buenos Aires, Argentina
Stefan Seregard, MD, Stockholm, Sweden
Roger Macklis, MD, Cleveland, Ohio, USA

Singh AD, Pelayes DE, Seregard S, Macklis R (eds): Ophthalmic Radiation Therapy. Techniques and Applications.
Dev Ophthalmol. Basel, Karger, 2013, vol 52, pp 1–14 (DOI: 10.1159/000351045)

Introduction to Radiotherapy and Standard Teletherapy Techniques

Ehsan H. Balagamwala[a] · Abigail Stockham[a] · Roger Macklis[a] · Arun D. Singh[b]

[a]Department of Radiation Oncology, Taussig Cancer Institute and [b]Department of Ophthalmic Oncology, Cole Eye Institute, Cleveland Clinic Foundation, Cleveland, Ohio, USA

Abstract

Radiation was first discovered in the late 19th century by Wilhelm Roentgen and has since been used extensively to treat a variety of cancers. Over the last century, we have developed an extensive understanding of the physical properties of radiation as well as radiation biology. Technological advances in the last few decades in medical imaging and radiotherapy delivery have led to the development of highly complex radiation delivery systems such as intensity modulated radiotherapy, which can be utilized to conformally treat complex tumor shapes while minimizing radiation dose to the surrounding normal tissue. To completely appreciate the application of radiotherapy for ophthalmic cancers, it is important to have a basic understanding of radiation therapy. In this chapter, we will discuss the fundamentals of radiation and radioactive decay, the mechanism of tumor cell damage leading to tumor cell apoptosis, as well as radiation and treatment parameters that are relevant for an ophthalmic oncologist. We will also discuss the concept of tissue tolerance which is of critical importance when prescribing radiation treatment as well as introduce the principles of three-dimensional conformal radiotherapy and intensity modulated radiotherapy.

Radiation was first described as 'X-rays' by Wilhelm Roentgen in 1895 while he was experimenting with the discharge of electricity in vacuum tubes. Henri Becquerel, Marie Curie and Pierre Curie built on the understanding of radiation a few months later when they described the emission of radiation by uranium [1]. These discoveries in the late 1890s and early 1900s not only revolutionized the scientific community's understanding of physics, but also medicine as X-rays were used to treat cancers as early as 1896. Soon after this external application of X-rays for therapeutic intervention, radon was implanted into tumors introducing the concept of brachytherapy. Advances over the last century have furthered radiation physics, radiation biology, and the therapeutic application of radiation in the management of ophthalmologic malignancies.

Each decade of the early 20th century ushered in new technological capabilities in radiation technology. Low-voltage X-ray machines, used the treatment of superficial malignancies, were introduced in the 1920s. In 1932, the first cyclotron was engineered at the University of California at Berkley, which led to the advent of charged particle radiotherapy. Further technological progress occurred in the 1950s with the development of the first cobalt-60 unit. Development of the cobalt-60 radiotherapy unit in 1951 was significant for both its eventual commercial availability and dosimetric characteristic of the averaged 1.25 MeV gamma rays emitted upon the decay of the radionuclide. During the same decade, another option for teletherapy was developed. The linear particle accelerator (linac) accelerates electrons, which allows for generation of megavoltage electron and photon beams, which are used in the treatment of ophthalmologic malignancies. The first modern high-energy linac was manufactured in Hammersmith Hospital in London in 1953 [2]. The first patient in the United States to undergo treatment with a linac was a 2-year-old boy with retinoblastoma, treated at Stanford Medical Center in 1956 [3].

In more recent decades, advancements in medical imaging, such as CT and MRI in the 1970s and 1980s, as well as patient immobilization, have led to the development of sophisticated and more precise radiation therapy techniques. Techniques such three-dimensional conformal radiation therapy (3D-CRT), intensity modulated radiotherapy (IMRT) developed in parallel in the 1990s and early 2000s. Over this same period of time, stereotactic radiosurgery (SRS), which was first developed in 1953, was modernized with the GammaKnife® [4] and linac-based SRS was pioneered. All of these techniques allow therapeutic quantities of energy deposition and absorption to a defined target, while minimizing damage to normal surrounding tissue. This chapter will focus on reviewing the basic principles of radiation therapy and standard radiotherapy techniques, such as 3D-CRT and IMRT, used in external beam radiotherapy. The next chapter will continue the current discussion with an introduction to more advanced radiotherapy techniques, including SRS and heavy ion therapy. Brachytherapy will then be discussed in the next two chapters.

Basic Principles of Radiotherapy

The unique characteristics of each element are a function of its atomic structure, i.e. the number and configuration of electrons, protons and neutrons. The atom is held together by strong subatomic bonds. When these bonds are disrupted, energy is released. This may occur as a result of external radiation or may occur when an atom undergoes radioactive decay. Radiation is the propagation of this energy through space or matter. It can take the form of electromagnetic waves, energetic particles or both. Radiotherapy exerts is effect on tissues as a result of the interaction between ra-

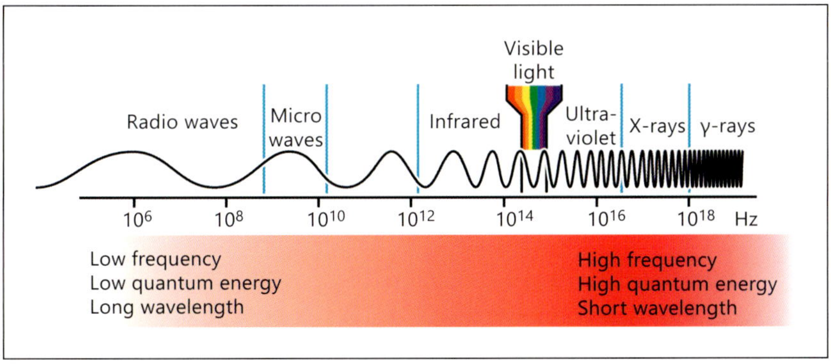

Fig. 1. The electromagnetic spectrum. High-frequency, small wavelength radiation is utilized in radiotherapy to treat tumors. Depending on the energy of the radiation, it can be optimized for diagnostic imaging versus use for therapeutics.

diation and molecular composition of living cells. When radiation is of sufficient energy it can break chemical bonds between molecules, which generates ions and free radicals. These, in turn, induce damage by oxidizing DNA and other cellular contents critical for the viability and/or replication of cells [5].

Dual Nature of Radiation

Radiation can be in the form of electromagnetic waves, particles or both.

Electromagnetic Radiation

Electromagnetic (EM) radiation is a form of energy that exhibits wave-like behavior as it travels through space. Energy is transmitted at the speed of light (c), with an inverse relationship between the wavelength (λ) and frequency (ν): $c = \nu\lambda$. EM radiation has a broad range of wavelengths ranging from 10^{-13} m (ultra-high-energy X-rays) to 10^{7} m (radio waves). Visible light constitutes a very small band on the EM spectrum: 4×10^{-7} to 7×10^{-7} m (fig. 1). As the wavelength gets shorter, EM radiation gains the ability to ionize particles. Photons generated by linacs for use in radiotherapy have wavelengths in the range of 10^{-11} to 10^{-13} m [6].

Particle Radiation

Particle radiation refers to the energy carried by subatomic particles such as negatively charged electrons, positively charged protons, and uncharged neutrons. These particles are accelerated in either linacs (electrons) or cyclotrons (protons and neutrons) to clinically relevant energies. Upon introduction into a medium, they impart their energy to that medium in a manner specific to the characteristics of the particle beam and the medium [6].

Radioactive Decay
Certain naturally occurring and synthetic elements exist in a high-energy, unstable state. These elements transform to a more stable, low energy state through a process called *decay*. The excess energy is energy is emitted in the form of radiation. Multiple types of radiation can be emitted during radioactive decay. The three most clinically relevant type of radiation include positively charged alpha particles (helium nucleus), negatively charged beta particles (electrons) or electrically neutral gamma-rays. An important parameter in radioactive decay is half-life ($T_{1/2}$). The $T_{1/2}$ of a radioactive source is the time required for half the source to decay and is unique to each radionuclide. For a selected radionuclide, the treatment time increases as the source decays. The $T_{1/2}$ and the radiotherapeutic characteristics intrinsic to each radionuclide may influence which radionuclide is selected for a particular clinical therapy. Radioactive decay is utilized in cobalt-60 teletherapy units, GammaKnife radiosurgery (GKRS) and brachytherapy [6]. A variety of other radioactive sources are utilized in radiotherapy, most commonly utilized in brachytherapy. Brachytherapy refers to placement of a radiation source within or close to the tumor.

Ionizing and Nonionizing Radiation

When radiation passes through a medium, energy can be transferred from incident form of radiation to the atoms that compose the medium. Transfer of energy can result in both ionizing and nonionizing effects. Only ionizing radiation is clinically relevant. Ionization occurs when a neutral atom or molecule acquires a positive or negative charge, most frequently as a result of ejection of electrons. These ions interact with cellular components, including DNA, which affect cellular function and mitosis. Ionizing effects tend to dominate when higher energy (i.e. short wavelengths) radiation is utilized [5].

Mechanism of Radiation-Induced Cellular Damage

The most well-understood target of ionizing radiation is DNA. DNA damage, with subsequent cellular dysfunction and mitotic inhibition, occurs as a result of direct damage, indirect damage, or a combination of direct and indirect damage. Direct DNA damage refers to interaction between the incident form of radiation and cellular DNA, which results in single- or double-strand breaks which impair cellular function and preclude replication. This results in permanent senescence, cell death, or mitotic catastrophe and inability to replicate. Direct DNA damage predominates when large particle radiation, i.e. protons or alpha particles, is utilized (fig. 2) [5].

Indirect DNA damage is mediated by the formation of hydroxyl ions by radiation which, in turn, create DNA strand breaks. Hydroxyl ions are generated when radia-

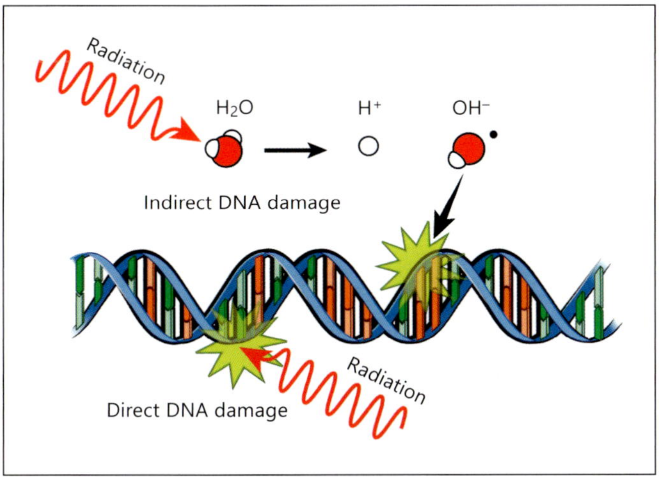

Fig. 2. Direct and indirect DNA damage in response to irradiation. Direct action dominates for more densely ionizing radiations, such as neutrons, because the secondary charged particles produced (protons, α-particles, and heavier nuclear fragments) result in a dense column of ionizations more likely to interact with the DNA. Indirect DNA damage via OH^- ions dominates when less dense ionizing radiation such as photons or gamma rays are utilized.

tion overcomes the binding energy of the hydrogen and oxygen molecules of water, resulting in hydroxyl and oxygen ions. Indirect DNA damage predominates when photons or electrons are utilized.

Teletherapy Sources

Teletherapy, contemporarily referred to as external beam radiotherapy, denotes delivery of radiation from an external source at a distance. In modern clinical radiation oncology, a linear accelerator or a cyclotron is used to generate and deliver external beam photon or particle radiotherapy. While it may be used for standard teletherapy, cobalt-60 is most frequently utilized as a part of the GKRS system.

Cobalt-60 Unit

A cobalt-60 unit houses a radioactive cobalt source that emits gamma-radiation as cobalt-60 decays to nickel-60. Cobalt-60 has a $T_{1/2}$ of 5.27 years. As the source ages, the quantity remaining in the cobalt-60 state versus the nickel-60 state declines, thus, the time required to deliver a certain amount of radiation increases. The average energy of the γ photon beam is 1.25 MeV. In modern practice, cobalt-60 is most often utilized as part of the GKRS system, which houses 201 cobalt-60 sources targeted at a single point (fig. 3). GKRS is one form of stereotactic radiosurgery utilized for the management of ophthalmic tumors.

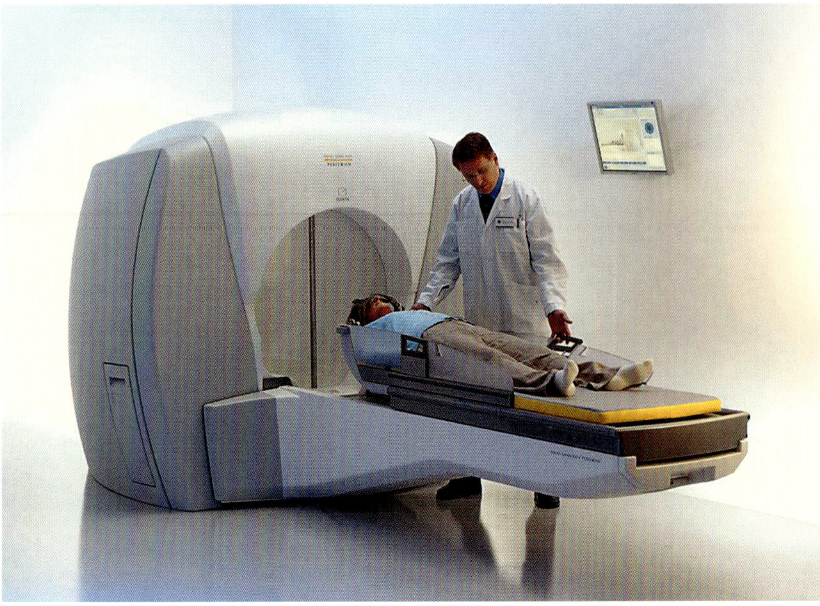

Fig. 3. GammaKnife radiosurgery. This radiotherapy system utilizes 201 Cobalt-60 sources which emit gamma rays, all focused to a single point. Image courtesy of Elekta, Inc.

Linear Accelerator

A linear accelerator (fig. 4) uses high-frequency electromagnetic waves to accelerate charged particles, most often electrons, to high energies (MeV) through a linear vacuum tube. This monoenergetic electron beam can be utilized to treat superficial tumors (see 'Depth Dose' under 'Radiation Parameters') or can be directed to a target (typically tungsten). This interaction between electrons and tungsten generates high energy X-rays, called photons. A uniform 6 MeV electron beam generates photons with a maximum energy of 6 MeV, while the 'average' energy is approximately one-third of the maximum energy, or 2 MeV. The higher the energy of the electron beam, the higher the energy of the resultant photons. The energy of the electron beam, and the resultant photon beam, can be adjusted based on the medical application desired. Generally, electron beams are used to treat superficial tumors and photon beams are used to spare the skin while providing adequate dose a depth to treat deeper tumors. The primary advantages of a linear accelerator over a single cobalt-60 source are the higher dose rate, more uniform dose distribution, no radioactive source, and the ability to generate both electron and photon beams with different energies [6].

Cyclotron

In contrast to linacs, which are used to accelerate light particles such as electrons, a cyclotron is used to accelerate heavy particles such as protons and neutrons. Protons effect direct DNA damage as they traverse biological tissue. The use of protons in radiation

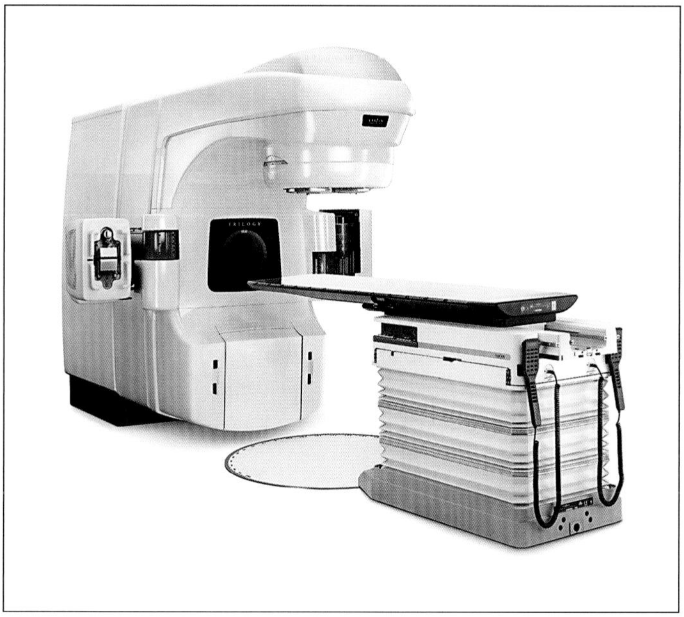

Fig. 4. A linear accelerator or 'Linac' emits either electrons or photons for use in radiotherapy. Image courtesy of Varian Medical Systems, Inc. All rights reserved.

oncology has become more popular in recent years because of their physical dose distribution characteristic, called the Bragg peak. This refers to the steep peak of maximal dose deposit followed by a steep dose drop-off. A Bragg peak can be targeted to the tumor whilst maximally sparing the surrounding normal tissue [6]. The utility of protons is maximal in pediatric patients in whom life expectancy is the longest. Proton beam radiotherapy has been extensively utilized for the treatment of uveal melanomas [see chapter 'Radiation Therapy: Uveal Tumors' by Seregard et al., this vol.] as well as retinoblastoma [see chapter 'Radiation Therapy: Retinal Tumors' by Sethi et al., this vol.].

Radiation Parameters

Radiation Dose

An absorbed dose of radiation, commonly referred to as 'dose', is measured in grays. 1 Gy represents 1 J of energy absorbed by 1 kg mass. Historically, radiation dose was referred to as radiation absorbed dose, or 'rad', the units of which correspond to hundredths of a gray, or a centigray.

Depth Dose

As photons and electrons traverse through matter, their energy is attenuated by interactions with the medium. Attenuation depends on characteristics of the photon or particle beam and the unique composition of the attenuating matter. A depth-dose curve is an illustration of radiation attenuation as it passes through matter. Electrons tend to deposit their energy superficially, with 80–100% of the maximum absorbed dose delivered to the surface of the patient. Electronic equilibrium, which denotes maximum dose delivered, for electron beams varies from approximately 1–3 cm, depending on the energy of the electron beam. A relatively steep dose drop-off beyond the maximum depth occurs (fig. 5a). Photons demonstrate complementary characteristics to electrons in that they are more penetrating and tend to deliver the maximum dose to a depth of 2–4 cm, depending on the energy of the photon beam. Photons demonstrate a shallower dose drop-off compared to electrons (fig. 5b). Protons can have maximum dose at a variety of depths, depending on the energy of the proton beam. The deposition of energy over a short distance at the end of the particle's range in matter is called the Bragg peak. Beyond the Bragg peak, very little dose is deposited. The Bragg peak can be modified for the treatment of tumors of a variety of depths and sizes (fig. 5c) [6].

Relative Biological Effectiveness

As explained above, gray is a measure of energy absorbed per unit mass of tissue. As we have discussed above, different types of radiation lead to different biological effects. Therefore, equal doses of different types of radiation do not have equal biological responses. To compare the effectiveness of different types of radiation, relative biological effectiveness has been defined which is a ratio of the biologic effect of doses (D) of test radiation, r, and standard radiation, s, to produce an equivalent response (i.e. relative biological effectiveness = D_r/D_S). As shown in table 1, protons have a greater biological effectiveness than photons or electrons, owing to the characteristics of the interactions with the matter onto which they are incident [5].

Treatment Parameters

Target Volume

Several factors are considered when determining the volume of disease that must be treated with radiation: the volume of visible tumor, knowledge of the natural progression of disease on a population and individual level, error in accuracy of daily patient setup (including organ motion), and known errors in the accuracy of radiation beam targeting. The initial volume that is defined is called the gross tumor volume (GTV), which refers to the visible tumor volume based on imaging studies. Next, the clinical target volume (CTV) is defined which is an expansion of the GTV to account for microscopic disease based on our understanding of the natural progression of disease. The planning target volume (PTV) is an expansion of the CTV and takes into account the inaccuracies of daily patient set-up, organ motion, as well as beam targeting. Typically, a margin of 0.5–2.0 cm is added to the GTV to form the

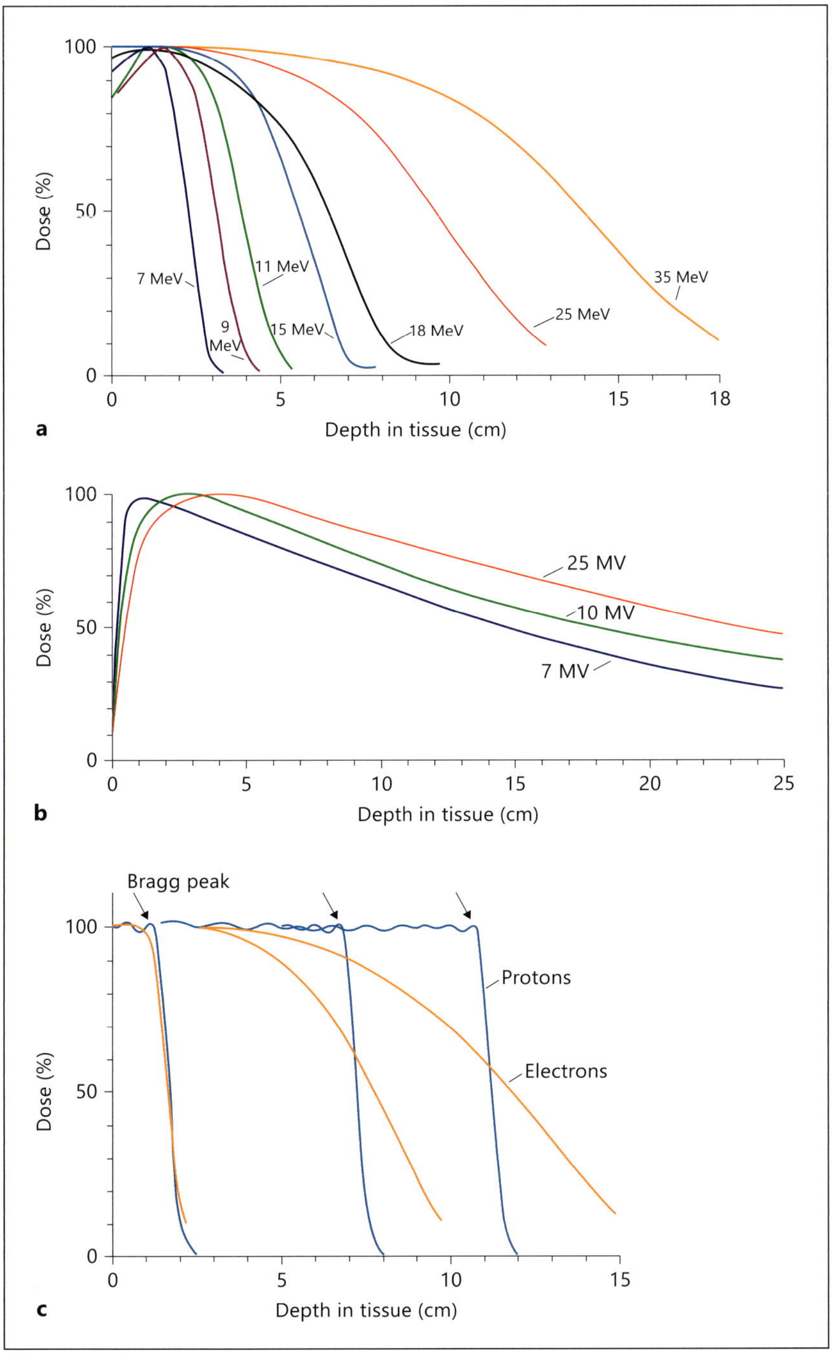

Fig. 5. Depth dose curve showing the dose distribution of different energies at different tissue depths. **a** Electrons. **b** Photons. **c** Protons. Modified from Khan [6].

Table 1. Relative biological effectiveness values of commonly used radiations

Radiation	Relative biological effectiveness
Standard (250 kVp X-rays)	1.0
Linac (6–15 MeV)	~0.8
Cobalt-60	0.8–0.9
Protons	~1.1
Neutrons (19 MeV)	1–2

Reproduced with permission from Anderson C, Fleming P, Wilkinson A, Singh AD: Principles of radiation therapy; in Singh, Damato, Pe'er, Murphree, Perry (eds): Clinical Ophthalmic Oncology. Amsterdam, Elsevier Saunders, 2007.

PTV and the radiation dose is prescribed to the PTV. The size of the PTV varies based on anticipated organ motion, reproducibility of daily set-up, and use of image-guided radiation therapy.

Total Dose

The most important factors considered when determining total radiation dose are the responsiveness of the tumor to radiation and surrounding normal tissue tolerance. Other factors considered include the purpose of radiation (curative versus palliative) as well as whether gross disease is present or only microscopic disease (i.e. postsurgical resection).

Fractionation

In general, conventional external beam radiation treatments require that the total radiation dose be divided into fractions delivered over several weeks in order to avoid toxicity. Fractionation allows normal tissue to undergo repair with greater efficacy than tumor cells, secondary to faulty repair mechanisms. With the advent of advanced immobilization techniques and the ability to perform stereotactic radiosurgery, select patients can be treated in a single fraction, thereby potentially maximizing tumor control whilst sparing normal tissue toxicity.

Toxicity can be divided into two groups: acute and late toxicity. Acute toxicity is directly correlated with total dose whereas late toxicity is correlated with dose per fraction. The larger the dose per fraction, the higher the risk of developing late toxicity, such as severe dry eye, cataract or optic neuropathy. On the other hand, the smaller the dose per fraction, the lower the therapeutic effects of radiation, i.e. tumor kill. Most conventional fractionation schemes utilize a dose of 180–200 cGy administered 5 days per week, though data suggest that hyperfractionation (110–120 cGy twice daily) reduces the risk of radiation retinopathy in patients treated for head and neck cancers [7]. Palliative radiation therapy tends to utilize higher doses per fraction with the assumption that the natural course of disease will preclude the development of later radiation toxicity. Some commonly reported dose fractionation schemes for ocular cancers are shown in table 2.

Table 2. External beam radiation therapy dose/fractionation schedules for common ophthalmic cancers

Disease	Total dose	Dose per fraction	Number of fractions
Uveal melanoma	60–70 CGE (protons)	14–15 CGE	4–5
Retinoblastoma	40–50 Gy	2–2.5 Gy	20–25
Uveal/orbital metastasis	40 Gy	2 Gy	20
Orbital lymphoma	30 Gy	2 Gy	15
Basal or squamous cell carcinoma of the eyelid	35–42.5 Gy	4.25–7 Gy	5–10
Palliation	30 Gy	3 Gy	10

CGE = Cobalt gray equivalent.

Table 3. Normal tissue tolerance dose to external beam radiation (cGy)

Organ	Complication rate at 5 years		Clinical endpoint
	5%	50%	
Brain	6,000	7,500	necrosis, infarction
Optic nerve	5,000	6,500	visual acuity <20/200
Optic chiasm	5,000	6,500	visual acuity <20/200
Lens	1,000	1,800	symptomatic cataract
Retina	4,500	6,500	visual acuity <20/200

Reproduced with permission from Anderson C, Fleming P, Wilkinson A, Singh AD: Principles of radiation therapy; in Singh, Damato, Pe'er, Murphree, Perry (eds): Clinical Ophthalmic Oncology. Amsterdam, Elsevier Saunders, 2007.

Tissue Tolerance

Strong knowledge of the spectrum of potential complications for radiotherapy and established parameters for avoidance of complications is imperative. When planning ocular radiotherapy, the most important normal structures include the lens, retina, optic nerve, optic chiasm, opposite orbit, pituitary and the brain. The tolerance parameters of these structures vary based on whether the patient will undergo conventionally fractionated radiotherapy, or undergo stereotactic radiosurgery. When planning radiation treatments, it also important to consider patient factors such as prior, concurrent, or future chemotherapy administration, age, and comorbidities such as diabetes, which can alter normal tissue tolerance. Table 3 details the normal tissue tolerance to conventionally fractionated (180–200 cGy/fraction) external beam radiation [8]. For a more detailed analysis of tissue tolerance, we refer the interested reader to recently published meta-analysis [9, 10]. A detailed discussion of ophthalmic complications of radiotherapy can be found elsewhere in this book [see chapters 'Radiation Therapy: Anterior Segment Complications' by Medina Mendez and Singh and 'Radiation Therapy: Posterior Segment Complications' by Seregard et al., this vol.].

Teletherapy Techniques

Simulation and Treatment Planning
Prior to initiation of radiotherapy planning and administration, patients complete appropriate ophthalmologic evaluation, diagnostic imaging, and are seen in consultation by a radiation oncologist. Based on the clinicoradiographic scenario, the multidisciplinary team can develop the appropriate treatment plan. When the team and radiation oncologist deem external beam radiotherapy to be appropriate, the first step in the treatment process is for the patient to undergo simulation of radiotherapy. Simulation refers to a several-step process. First, the patient is placed in the treatment position using an immobilization device, such as a thermoplastic mask. Next, the patient undergoes a CT scan in the treatment position to define the clinical anatomy. The target volume and nearby critical anatomic structures are defined on the simulation CT images. Often, this is completed with MRI coregistration to aid in target delineation. Physicians determine the appropriate treatment volumes, definition of critical structures, constraints on critical structures. Medical dosimetrists assign a beam arrangement and direct the treatment planning system over a series of iterations to generate an optimal treatment plan, balancing adequate treatment of the target while achieving dose-constraints designed to minimize treatment toxicity. In order to reduce dose to the lens, several lens-sparing beam arrangements have been devised (table 4) [11–18]. Once the individualized treatment plan has been devised, the physician reviews it and medical physicists ensure quality assurance by comparing actual radiation delivery versus anticipated radiation delivery.

Three-Dimensional Conformal Radiotherapy
Prior to the availability of CT or MRI imaging, bony landmarks were utilized to assist in radiation field planning. However, with the advent of advanced imaging modalities, it is possible to define the treatment target in three dimensions. Thus, 3D-CRT was possible. Using CT simulation images, the therapeutic target and associated normal tissues are appreciated in three dimensions and identified. Radiation beams can then be arranged in order to achieve maximal target volume coverage while maximally avoiding normal structures. This is possible using multileaf collimators, which allow shaping the radiation beam to be as conformal, or similarly shaped, to the tumor as possible. Once the radiation fields are arranged, advanced algorithms can be used to measure the dose to each contoured structure including the target volume and normal structures. Amongst other advantages over two-dimensional planning, 3D-CRT allows for objective comparison of 3D dose distributions between several treatment

Table 4. Lens-sparing techniques for external beam radiation therapy

Technique	Year	Author
Direct lateral field posterior to the lens	1977	Chu et al. [11]
	1982	Brady et al. [12]
	1994	Nylen et al. [13]
Oblique lateral field with lens shielding	1977	Chu et al. [11]
	1977	Maor et al. [14]
Anterior field with lens block	1977	Chu et al. [11]
Right-angled wedged fields	1982	Brady et al. [12]
Direct lateral field with D shape block	1983	Schipper [15]
Proton beam therapy	1983	Goitein [17]
Oblique electron fields with lens block	1997	Steenbakkers et al. [17]
Modified Schipper technique	2003	Bajcsay et al. [18]

Reproduced with permission from Anderson C, Fleming P, Wilkinson A, Singh AD: Principles of radiation therapy; in Singh, Damato, Pe'er, Murphree, Perry (eds): Clinical Ophthalmic Oncology. Amsterdam, Elsevier Saunders, 2007.

plans. The process of first arranging radiation fields and then calculating the dose distribution is termed forward planning. All 2D planning was forward-planned in that radiation dosimetrists and physicists applied known beam arrangements and manually adjusted collimator leaves and beam weighting over several iterations to achieve an optimal plan.

Intensity Modulated Radiation Therapy

IMRT is an advanced type of high-precision radiotherapy that is the next generation of 3D-CRT. IMRT utilizes inverse planning, which means that the desired dose distribution criteria are set prior to determining the optimal beam arrangements. Computer algorithms in advanced treatment planning software systems generate beam arrangements to meet the required dose distribution criteria. The principle of IMRT is to target the tumor using multiple nonuniform beams, which have been optimized to maximally irradiate the target while minimizing radiation to the surrounding normal structures. IMRT utilizes multi-leaf collimators, which allows shaping of the beam to conform to complex target shapes such as when the tumor wraps around a critical structure. IMRT also enables modulation of the radiation beam such that the intensity of the radiation dose is highest within the tumor (i.e. the tumor is 'hot') whilst the intensity in critical structures is the lowest (i.e. critical structures are 'cold'). This is done by the treatment planning software, which divides the radiation beam into a large number of beamlets and determines the optimal intensity of each beamlet to meet dose distribution criteria. Modulation of the radiation beam intensity and dynamic shaping of the radiation beam are the differentiating factors between IMRT and 3D-CRT.

Conclusion

Over the last half century, radiotherapy has undergone significant technological and biological advancements. The advent of IMRT and image-guided radiation therapy has allowed for increased conformity of radiotherapy dose delivery to target volume while sparing surrounding normal tissue, with resultant improvements in toxicity and ambitions of increasing local control. Advances in the basic science of radiation-induced DNA damage have allowed for the development of mathematical models to compare different radiation dose and fractionation schemes. Significant strides have been made in the use of a variety of radiotherapy techniques to achieve improving local control of ophthalmic tumors while minimizing toxicity. Further technological and scientific breakthroughs will allow for greater understanding of the biology of ophthalmologic pathology and novel radiotherapeutic interventions to optimize oncologic outcomes and patient quality of life. The basic terminology and radiotherapeutic concepts discussed will be developed further in the following chapters of this book.

References

1 Lederman M: The early history of radiotherapy: 1895–1939. Int J Radiat Oncol Biol Phys 1981;7:639–648.
2 Thwaites DI, Tuohy JB: Back to the future: the history and development of the clinical linear accelerator. Phys Med Biol 2006;51:R343–R362.
3 Jones H, Illes J, Northway W: A history of the Department of Radiology at Stanford University. AJR Am J Roentgenol 1995;164:753–760.
4 Leksell L: The stereotaxic method and radiosurgery of the brain. Acta Chir Scand 1951;102:316–319.
5 Hall EJ, Giaccia AJ: Radiobiology for the Radiologist. Philadelphia, Wolters Kluwer Health/Lippincott Williams & Wilkins, 2012.
6 Khan FM: The Physics of Radiation Therapy. Philadelphia, Lippincott Williams & Wilkins, 2010.
7 Monroe AT, Bhandare N, Morris CG, Mendenhall WM: Preventing radiation retinopathy with hyperfractionation. Int J Radiat Oncol Biol Phys 2005;61:856–864.
8 Emami B, Lyman J, Brown A, et al: Tolerance of normal tissue to therapeutic irradiation. Int J Radiat Oncol Biol Phys 1991;21:109–122.
9 Lawrence YR, Li XA, el Naqa I, et al: Radiation dose-volume effects in the brain. Int J Radiat Oncol Biol Phys 2010;76:S20–S27.
10 Mayo C, Martel MK, Marks LB, et al: Radiation dose-volume effects of optic nerves and chiasm. Int J Radiat Oncol Biol Phys 2010;76:S28–S35.
11 Chu FC, Huh SH, Nisce LZ, Simpson LD: Radiation therapy of choroid metastasis from breast cancer. Int J Radiat Oncol Biol Phys 1977;2:273–279.
12 Brady LW, Shields JA, Augsburger JJ, Day JL: Malignant intraocular tumors. Cancer 1982;49:578–585.
13 Nylén U, Kock E, Lax I, et al: Standardized precision radiotherapy in choroidal metastases. Acta Oncol 1994;33:65–68.
14 Maor M, Chan RC, Young SE: Radiotherapy of choroidal metastases: breast cancer as primary site. Cancer 1977;40:2081–2086.
15 Schipper J: An accurate and simple method for megavoltage radiation therapy of retinoblastoma. Radiother Oncol 1983;1:31–41.
16 Goitein M, Miller T: Planning proton therapy of the eye. Med Phys 1983;10:275–283.
17 Steenbakkers RJ, Altschuler MD, D'Angio GJ, et al: Optimized lens-sparing treatment of retinoblastoma with electron beams. Int J Radiat Oncol Biol Phys 1997;39:589–594.
18 Bajcsay A, Kontra G, Récsán Z, et al: Lens-sparing external beam radiotherapy of intraocular metastases: our experiences with twenty four eyes. Neoplasma 2003;50:459–464.

Abigail Stockham, MD
Department of Radiation Oncology
Cleveland Clinic Foundation
9500 Euclid Ave, T-28, Cleveland, OH 44195 (USA)
E-Mail stockha@ccf.org

Singh AD, Pelayes DE, Seregard S, Macklis R (eds): Ophthalmic Radiation Therapy. Techniques and Applications.
Dev Ophthalmol. Basel, Karger, 2013, vol 52, pp 15–28 (DOI: 10.1159/000351050)

Teletherapy: Advanced Techniques

Abigail Stockham[a] · Ehsan H. Balagamwala[a] · Arun D. Singh[b] · Roger Macklis[a]

[a]Department of Radiation Oncology, Taussig Cancer Institute, and [b]Department of Ophthalmic Oncology, Cole Eye Institute, Cleveland Clinic Foundation, Cleveland, Ohio, USA

Abstract

Radiotherapy has been utilized as a treatment for ophthalmologic processes for more than one hundred years. Over this century, the field of ophthalmologic oncology has been revolutionized through medical discoveries, development of novel surgical interventions, and innovation of advanced radiotherapy techniques. In this chapter, novel radiotherapy techniques are considered. Material presented will build on basic radiation therapy principles, techniques, and treatment parameters established in the previous chapter through consideration of intensity modulated radiotherapy, stereotactic radiotherapy, and heavy ion therapy. Deliberation of matters common across advanced radiotherapy techniques including target delineation, treatment planning, and requisites for ensuring accurate, precise treatment delivery will precede discussion of advanced radiotherapy techniques as applied to the management ophthalmologic malignancies.

Radiotherapy has played an integral role in the management of ocular tumors since the early 20th century. The use of teletherapy, or external beam radiotherapy, was reported as early as 1902 and the application of radium published reports on the application of radium for the management of ocular pathology was reported by 1905 [1–3]. Progress in engineering over the first half of the 20th century resulted in development of the linear accelerator and treatment of the first patient in the Western Hemisphere with a linear accelerator, a vision-sparing therapeutic intervention for a small child with retinoblastoma [4]. While linear accelerators remain the most-widely used delivery system in modern radiotherapy, the intervening six decades of research have resulted in development of advanced teletherapy techniques including intensity modulated radiotherapy (IMRT), stereotactic radiosurgery, fractionated stereotactic radiation therapy, and heavy particle ion therapy. As with the linear accelerator, ophthalmologic tumors were among the earliest and, to date, most well-studied indications for the utilization of heavy ion therapy [5–17].

Over the past several decades, progress in the fields of biology and physics have allowed for increasingly accurate identification of treatment target. Radiotherapy treatment planning computer software is capable of generating complex treatment plans in a timely fashion. Finally, sophisticated treatment delivery systems enable very precise treatment delivery. As a result, it is possible to deliver large quantities of radiation to small ophthalmologic targets while sparing nearby normal structures irradiation to tumoricidal doses.

Highly Conformal External Beam Radiation Therapy

Historically, radiotherapy utilized 2-dimensional fluoroscopic radiographs with field definition guided by bony anatomy. As the orbital contents are not well visualized on plane film radiographs, simple, standard field arrangements were often employed with generous fields to avoid treatment failure secondary to 'geographic miss'. Modern radiotherapy systems are capable of highly conformal external beam radiation therapy, whereby the volume of tissue receiving a therapeutic or prescribed dose of radiation very closely approximates what the physician has identified as the target volume. This is accomplished through accurate delineation of the target volume, utilization of modern treatment planning software, and imaging immediately prior to each treatment so as to confirm accurate alignment of the patient prior to treatment.

Identification of Target

Identification of the treatment target in ophthalmic malignancies has improved with the advent of cross sectional imaging methods such as computed tomography (CT) and magnetic resonance imaging (MRI). Prior to the availability of cross-sectional imaging, target delineation had been performed, with basic calculations and plain film radiographs. As such, only basic treatment fields, or portals, were feasible. In recent decades, treatment planning has changed significantly with through utilization of CT images for through the area target region. The physician will then identify the tumor and any areas at risk for microscopic tumor extension on each planning CT slice through a process called, 'segmentation'.

Acquisition of a planning CT scan not only allows for improved visualization of the gross tumor over plain films; CT scans provide important information for including electronic density of a medium, which informs the deposition of energy, or dose, for megavoltage photons. The orbital contents are often more clearly visualized with MRI imaging than CT imaging; however, simulators are not widely available. Therefore, diagnostic MRI images often are coregistered to the CT scan obtained during virtual simulation, which allows for optimizing both target delineation and dose distribution (fig. 1).

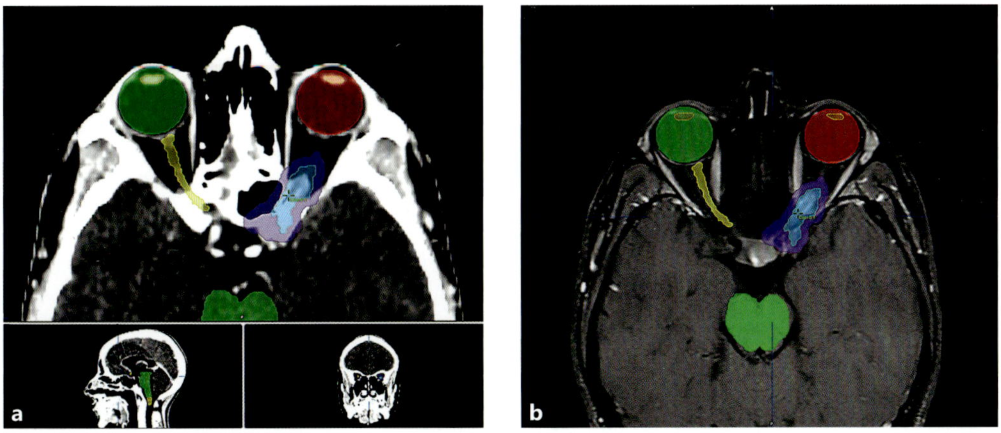

Fig. 1. Computed tomography (CT) scan for treatment planning (**a**) with MRI coregistration (**b**) denoting the gross tumor volume (blue) and planning target volume (purple). CT simulation confers optimization of geometric accuracy and it is on CT data that treatment planning algorithms are modeled. Reproduced with permission from Romanelli and Anschel: Radiosurgery for epilepsy. Lancet Neurol 2006;5:613–620. (http://www.sciencedirect.com/science/article/pii/S1474442206704963).

Treatment Planning

Treatment planning is an integral part of advanced teletherapy techniques for the treatment of ophthalmic malignancies. Treatment planning systems may be based on one or more mathematical models developed to predict relevant electromagnetic and particulate interactions for a given beam energy and medium. Summation of these interactions provides information regarding the distribution of energy absorbed by a medium, known as radiotherapy dose. Simple plans including one or two beams have been used in the management of ocular tumors for decades, but treatment planning software and contemporary delivery systems allow for plans with many beams of a variety of angles, intricate weighting of beams, and intensity modulation. Intensity modulation refers to nonuniform delivery of radiotherapy dose over a specified region. This allows for greater conformality of isodose distributions to treatment targets, sculpting distributions to avoid nearby critical structures, the potential for dose escalation and reduction of radiotherapy side effects (fig. 2) [18–20].

Image-Guided Radiation Therapy

Complex, conformal treatment plans are beneficial only when patient positioning is highly reproducible. For patients undergoing ocular radiotherapy, a thermoplastic mesh mask is commonly utilized to ensure the patient is properly positioned and maintenance of this position over the course of treatment. Once visual inspection of

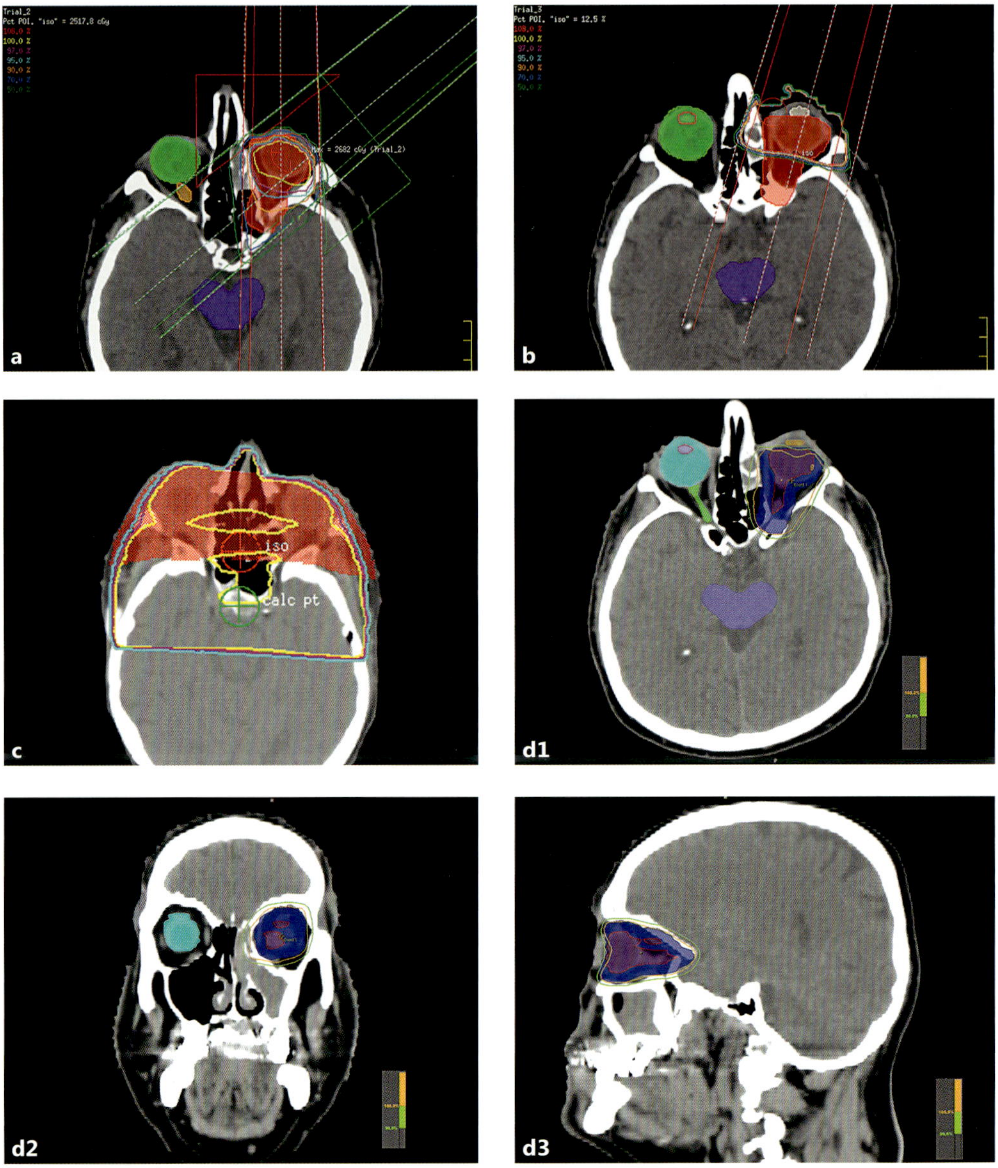

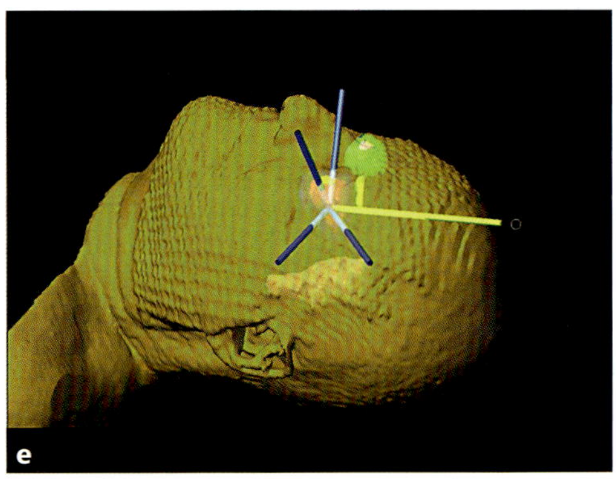

Fig. 2. Radiation therapy treatment plan for an orbital tumor using classic wedged-pair technique (**a**), electrons (**b**), opposed lateral fields (**c**), intensity-modulated radiation therapy (IMRT) axial (**d1**), coronal (**d2**), and sagittal (**d3**) 3-dimensional rendering, beam arrangement for IMRT (**e**). Reproduced with permission from Romanelli and Anschel: Radiosurgery for epilepsy. Lancet Neurol 2006;5:613–620. (http://www.sciencedirect.com/science/article/pii/S1474442206704963).

positioning is satisfactory, confirmation of positioning may be performed with image-guidance prior to treatment. Over the decades, many types of image-guidance have been developed. Before cross sectional imaging was available, plain radiographic portal images ('port films') were made to verify correct patient position and appropriate placement of blocks or field collimation.

Image guidance has undergone marked development in recent years. Current systems available include orthogonal imaging with planar radiographs, ultrasonography, cone-beam CT scans, fiducial markers with planar radiographs or cone-beam CT scans, radiofrequency transponders, infrared cameras, video cameras, and gating mechanisms that automatically can stop or resume treatment based on correct positioning of the patient or body part such as the eye (fig. 3) [21–24].

Optimization of image guidance techniques and real-time eye tracking during proton beam radiation therapy is needed to optimize dose delivery. Real-time videographic eye tracking may evaluate and help minimize eye movement during treatment; however, eye movement during treatment continues to be a problem that may limit the dose distribution advantages of proton beam radiation therapy [25–28]. Facial features may be extracted from MRI scans and transferred to software that uses input from an infrared camera to ensure that a patient is maintained in the treatment position.

Stereotactic Techniques

Stereotactic Methods

Stereotactic methods and image guidance are used in the treatment of ophthalmic malignancies. These techniques enable the delivery of high doses of radiation therapy, frequently in a small number of fractions, to a precise location such as an ophthalmic tumor. Stereotactic methods use physical coordinates determined from 3-dimensional imaging modalities such as MRI and CT scans, or physical measurements, to identify the location of a tumor and nearby normal structures in those three dimensions. To ensure the physical location or the tumor correctly aligns with the coordinates of the treatment planning system, a stereotactic frame and/or image guidance may be used. Currently available stereotactic radiotherapy delivery systems include the GammaKnife® (Elekta, Stockholm, Sweden), linac-based systems including CyberKnife®, or with charged particle therapy, such as proton therapy, delivered with cyclotron or synchrotron.

Stereotactic Radiosurgery (GammaKnife)

Stereotactic radiosurgery with the GammaKnife was pioneered by the Swedish neurosurgeon Lars Leksell in 1951 for the treatment of functional intracranial lesions such as trigeminal neuralgia [29]. This highly conformal technique uses the knowledge of an

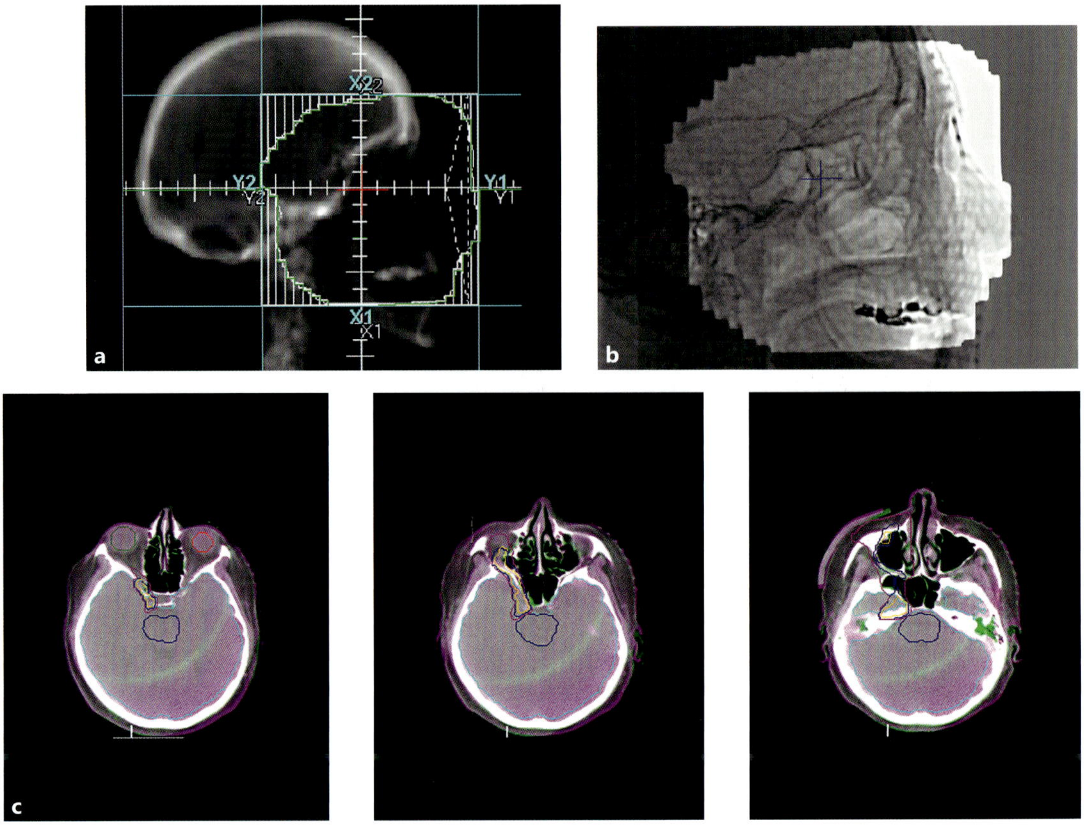

Fig. 3. Image guidance for highly conformal radiation therapy. **a** Patient position may be verified with portal images. Treatment portal imaging allows for rapid evaluation of proper alignment and placement of beam modifiers such as blocks and multi-leaf collimators. However, these images are of low-resolution and soft tissue visualization is poor. Reproduced with permission from http://www.sciencedirect.com/science/article/pii/S0360301610033237 – gr1. **b** Cone-beam CT provides improved resolution for visualization of the treatment target over portal imaging, but requires quality assurance to ensure the imaging center is correctly aligned to the isocenter of the linear accelerator, exposes the patient to greater quantities of radiotherapy for the purpose of image-guidance than portal imaging, and does not allow for intra-fraction image guidance. Beam modifiers such as blocks and multi-leaf collimators are not able to visualized with cone-beam CT. Reproduced with permission from http://www.sciencedirect.com/science/article/pii/S0360301611030070 – gr3. **c** Image guidance with high-resolution orthogonal radiographs allow for rapid, accurate evaluation of patient alignment in three dimensions and allows for intra-fraction image guidance, but volumetric information and soft tissue resolution is inferior to cone-beam CT. Reproduced with permission from: ExacTrac, Texas Oncology, Dallas Tex., USA. http://www.sciencedirect.com/science/article/pii/S095839470800040X – gr1.

anatomic structure or physical target in three coordinates, with reference to a surgically placed frame (fig. 4). The technique was initially developed with protons, but it is more practical to use numerous cobalt-60 sources that emit gamma rays [further discussed in the chapter 'Introduction to Radiotherapy and Standard Teletherapy Techniques' by Balagamwala et al., this vol.]. Stereotactic radiosurgery is favored frequently

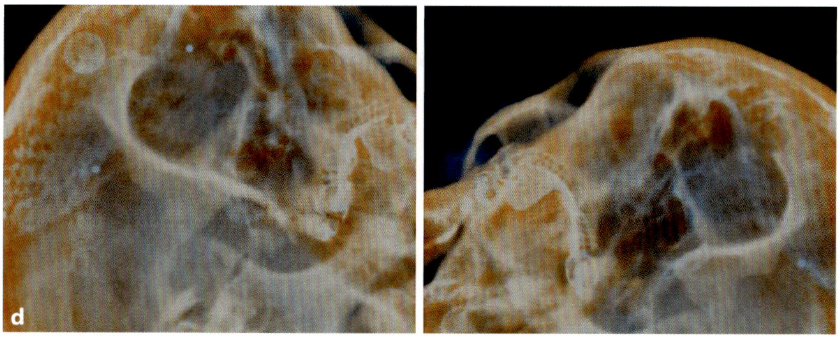

Fig. 3. Image guidance for highly conformal radiation therapy. **d** Video-based 3-dimensional optical surface imaging utilizes comparative reconstruction of real-time surface anatomy information to simulation CT surface. Reproduced with permission from Vision RT, Columbia, Md., USA.

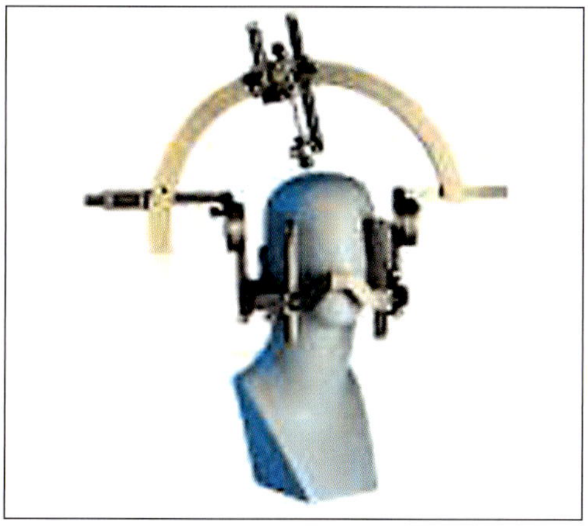

Fig. 4. Frame used in stereotactic radiosurgery (GammaKnife). The frame is attached to the patient's cranium. This rigid fixation ensures proper patient placement for delivery of highly conformal radiation therapy (d). Reproduced with permission from http://drkens.wordpress.com/2010/09/22/gamma-knife-therapy-for-brain-metastasis/dscn1667/.

because it may provide a highly conformal delivery of high doses of radiation therapy in a single session, with excellent local control and minimal adverse reactions [30–32].

Development of an optimal treatment plan with the GammaKnife starts with frame placement. A rigid metal frame is placed on the patient and attached to the skull at 4 points with pins, enabling immobilization and appropriate use of a localization system. A scalp-scaling device and planning CT scan are used, providing orientation and localization of the target in 3 dimensions. A high resolution volumetric MRI scan is obtained with slice thickness ≤1 mm, and the MRI scan is coregistered to the planning CT scan. Treatment planning is done in relation to spherical points ('shots') on the GammaKnife treatment planning system. For nonspherical targets, forward planning can be done to generate an isodose distribution conforming to the target.

Since the commercial development of the GammaKnife in the 1980s, this device has undergone several improvements. The recent model (GammaKnife® Perfexion

System) uses 192 sources of cobalt 60 with 24 independently controlled sectors and 3 collimator sizes (diameter: 4, 8 and 16 mm) that can be manipulated to conform to the shape of the treatment target (fig. 5).

After a treatment plan has been generated, the patient is brought to the treatment room. The treatment target is immobilized by attaching the frame to the treatment table. The physicians and physicists exit the room and the doors of the GammaKnife open. The automated table places the patient in the correct position determined in planning. Many small radiation beams are delivered, converging on the target with highly conformal ablative radiation doses. The duration of the treatment with GammaKnife stereotactic radiosurgery depends on the complexity of the target and the activity of the cobalt source.

GammaKnife stereotactic radiosurgery has been used in the treatment of ophthalmic malignancies including uveal melanoma, orbital paraganglioma, choroidal hemangiomas, cranial nerve schwannomas, and choroidal metastases [30, 33–38]. The effectiveness and adverse reactions are considered comparable between GammaKnife stereotactic radiosurgery, though dosimetric data suggests protons may confer a slightly decreased risk of second malignancies than photons when life expectancy is many decades [39–42].

Linear Accelerator-Based Stereotactic Radiosurgery

Linac-based stereotactic radiosurgery is similar in principle to GammaKnife stereotactic radiosurgery. However, with linac-based stereotactic radiosurgery, treatment is delivered with a linac and there is no radioactive source. Both standard linear accelerators and CyberKnife linear accelerators have are used in the delivery of stereotactic radiotherapy as part of the management of ophthalmologic malignancies [43–45].

Linac-based stereotactic radiosurgery may be delivered with or without a frame to position the patient. It frequently is performed with 6 MV photons that are generated when electrons, emitted from an electron gun, are accelerated through a waveguide to very high speeds; the electrons are directed at a target of high atomic number, usually tungsten, and undergo bremsstrahlung interactions to generate photons. The photon beam is collimated to a very small beam that delivers high conformal treatment to a small area such as the eye. Linac-based stereotactic radiosurgery typically is performed with a series of noncoplanar arcs.

The Cyberknife linac-based stereotactic radiosurgery system consists of a small, single energy linear accelerator mounted on a robotic arm (CyberKnife Robotic Radiosurgery System, Accuray, Sunnyvale, Calif., USA) (fig. 6). The robotic arm enables a wide range of potential treatment angles, and limitations from potential collisions between the treatment couch and gantry are avoided. Image guidance ensures correct alignment of the patient for optimal treatment delivery.

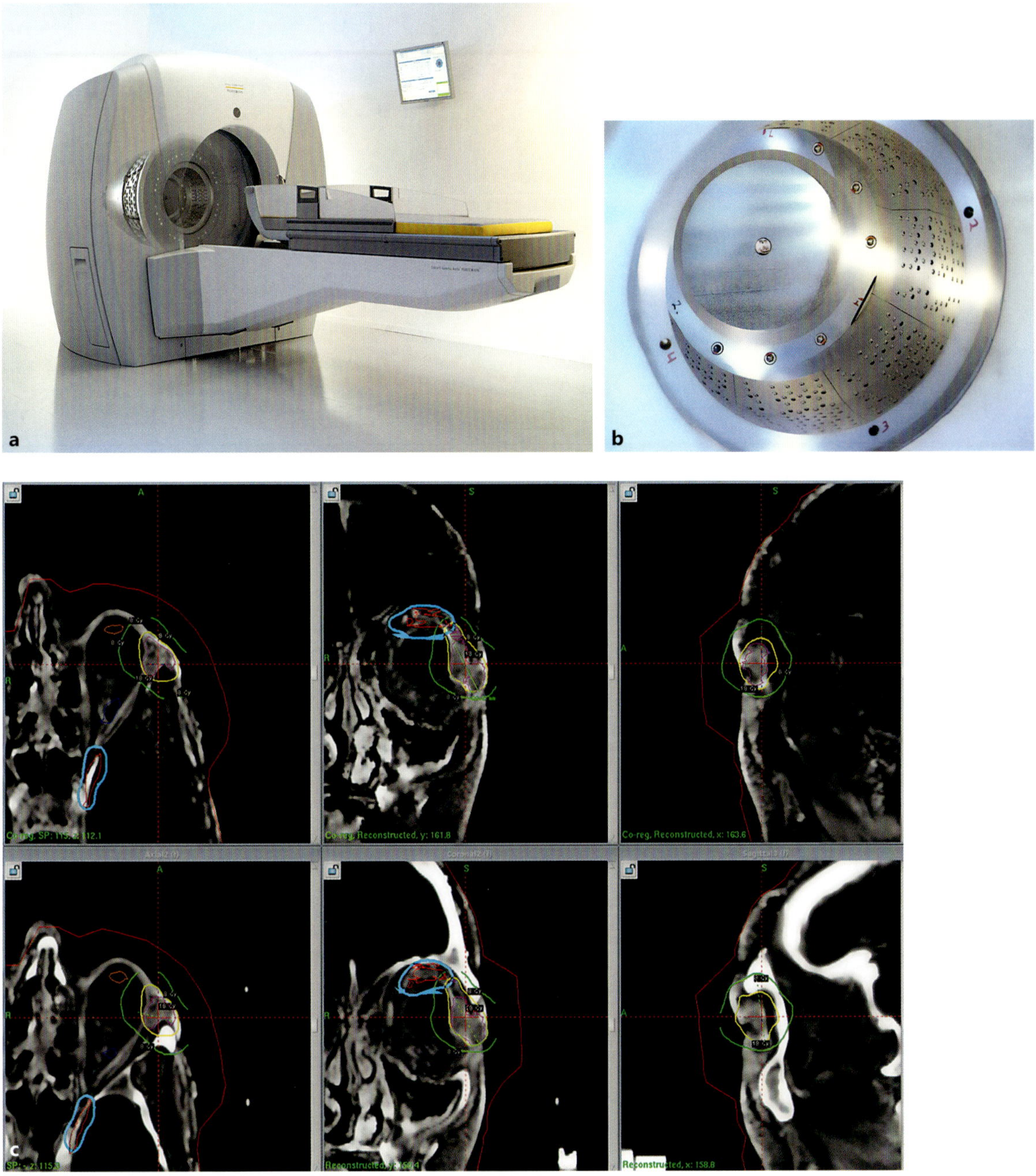

Fig. 5. The GammaKnife Perfexion system (**a**) has 192 sources of cobalt 60, with 24 sectors and various collimator sizes (4, 8, and 16 mm). The planning system uses the different sectors and collimator sizes (**b**) to create a highly conformal stereotactic radiosurgery treatment plan (**c**). Reproduced with permission from http://images.elektagallery.com/famain.asp?customerId = 476&sKey = 45ETMKVK&cid = 99 (**a** and **b**).

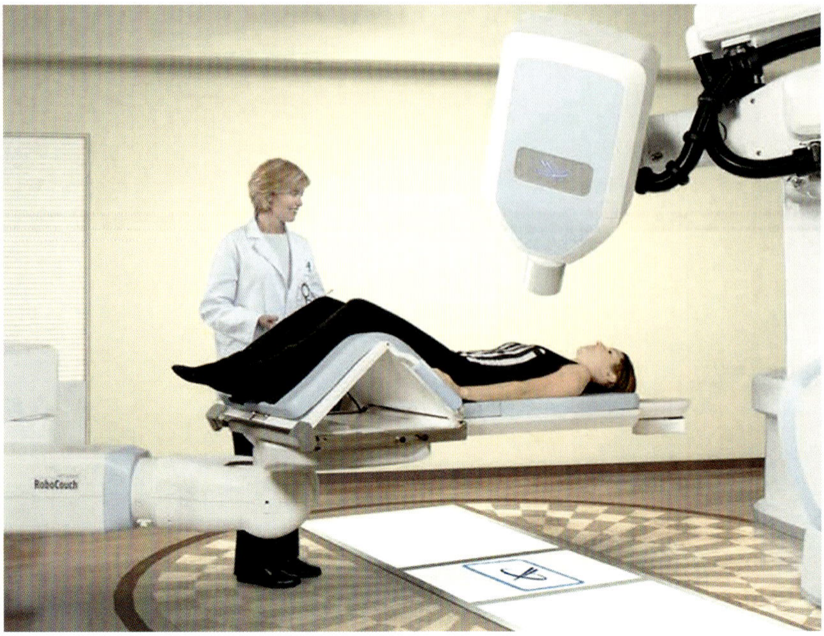

Fig. 6. A small, single energy linear accelerator mounted on an industrial robotic arm may be utilized for delivery of stereotactic radiotherapy (CyberKnife Robotic Radiosurgery System, Accuray). The robotic arm allows for greater freedom of movement. Image guidance is obtained through orthogonal planar radiographs. Reproduced with permission from http://www.cyberknife.com/uploadedFiles/CyberKnife_Overview/500929.A_CyberKnife_Patient_Brochure_FINAL.pdf.

Fractionated Stereotactic Radiation Therapy

Fractionated stereotactic radiation therapy uses the accurate anatomic precision available with GammaKnife and linac-based stereotactic radiosurgery. However, with fractionated stereotactic radiation therapy, the radiation is delivered over multiple treatments [43, 46–51].

Proton Therapy

Energy Distribution

The most common advanced teletherapy technique used in ophthalmic oncology is heavy ion therapy, including proton, carbon ion, and helium ion therapy. This therapy is possible because these ions are heavy and have an electric charge. The charge enables these ions to be accelerated in a cyclotron by rapidly alternating radiofrequency electric fields in a static magnetic field (fig. 7). The first cyclotron was engineered in Berkeley, Calif., USA, in 1932 [52].

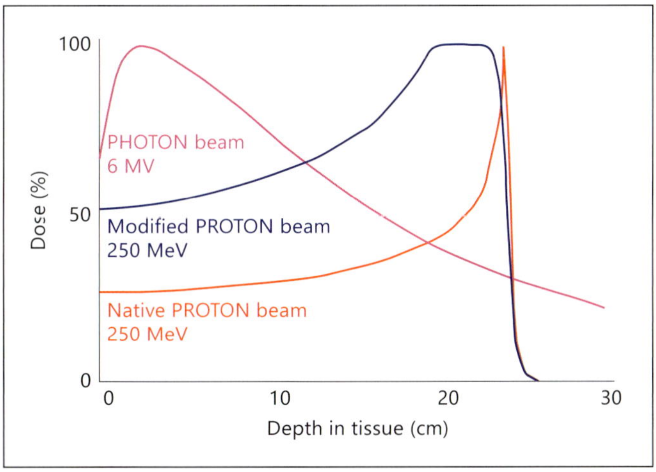

Fig. 7. A cyclotron is a circular device that accelerates charged particles to very high energies by rapidly alternating electrical fields in a static magnetic field. After the particles have been accelerated to the desired energy, they are siphoned off for collimation and delivery. Reproduced with permission from http://hyperphysics.phy-astr.gsu.edu/hbase/magnetic/cyclot.html.

Heavy ions have high linear energy transfer, and they are very effective at transferring energy to a surrounding medium. The Bragg peak [further discussed in the chapter 'Teletherapy: Standard Techniques' by Balagamwala et al., this vol.] refers to a low-entrance dose and deposition of a large amount of energy over a discrete region, with little energy deposition beyond the Bragg peak. Minimal dose deposition beyond the Bragg peak is particularly important in the treatment of ophthalmic tumors as critically important structures nearby may be at risk for radiation-induced damage, including the contralateral eye, brain and optic apparatus [53–58]. Although the physical dose distribution of protons, represented by the Bragg peak, offers the potential to minimize adverse effects on normal tissue, the narrow dose deposition of protons is a challenge for proton therapy for targets of sufficient depth or volume. A 'spread out Bragg peak' can be accomplished with a scanning proton beam or a series of repeated fields with different proton energies, allowing for dose deposition along a greater depth of tissue while sparing surrounding normal tissues [59, 60].

The proton beam can be focused using several techniques including spot scanning proton therapy and scattered proton therapy. In the past, proton beams had been shaped with poured or cut brass blocks for each proton field; this was cumbersome and required extensive time and space to cut and store these blocks. In recent years, spot scanning proton beam therapy has been developed, in which proton energies are changed for delivery of energy to varied depths of tissue. Although this avoids the need to cut or store brass blocks, spot scanning proton beam therapy may require a lengthy time of treatment when the proton energies are changed [61, 62].

Helium ion therapy has been used in the treatment of ophthalmic malignancies for >50 years. Helium ion therapy is similar to proton therapy because helium ions are heavily charged particles that have a prominent Bragg peak, optimal for treatment of smaller ophthalmic malignancies [63–68].

Conclusion

Advanced teletherapy techniques enable to delivery of highly conformal radiation therapy. These techniques may allow for dose escalation to treatment targets with decreased dose to nearby important structures to improve local control of ophthalmologic malignancies with reduced risk of normal tissue complications. Further developments are needed to optimize treatment delivery, including optimization of real-time image guidance with tracking or gating to improve the accuracy of dose delivery. Future treatments may be improved by the development of radiosensitizers, radioprotectants, altered dosing or fractionation schemes, gating technologies, and automated ocular recognition software.

References

1 Sweet W: Treatment of epithelioma of the eyelids by X-rays. Trans Am Ophthalmoll Soc 1902;9:540–545.
2 Manby A: Radium bromide in the treatment of rodent ulcer. Br Med J 1905;2:8–9.
3 Lawson A, Davidson JM: Radium therapy in eye disease. Br Med J 1910;2:1491–1497.
4 Ginzton EL, Nunan CS: History of microwave electron linear accelerators for radiotherapy. Int J Radiat Oncol Biol Phys 1985;11:205–216.
5 Finger PT: Radiation therapy for orbital tumors: concepts, current use, and ophthalmic radiation side effects. Surv Ophthalmol 2009;54:545–568.
6 Brada M, Pijls-Johannesma M, De Ruysscher D: Current clinical evidence for proton therapy. Cancer J 2009;15:319–324.
7 Brada M, Pijls-Johannesma M, De Ruysscher D: Proton therapy in clinical practice: current clinical evidence. J Clin Oncol 2007;25:965–970.
8 Bekkering GE, et al: The effectiveness and safety of proton radiation therapy for indications of the eye: a systematic review. Strahlenther Onkol 2009;185: 211–221.
9 Suit H, Urie M: Proton beams in radiation therapy. J Natl Cancer Inst 1992;84:155–164.
10 Gragoudas ES, et al: Proton irradiation of small choroidal malignant melanomas. Am J Ophthalmol 1977;83:665–673.
11 Gragoudas ES: Proton beam irradiation of uveal melanomas: the first 30 years. The Weisenfeld Lecture. Invest Ophthalmol Vis Sci 2006;47:4666–4673.
12 Gragoudas ES, et al: Proton beam irradiation. An alternative to enucleation for intraocular melanomas. Ophthalmology 1980;87:571–581.
13 Gragoudas ES, et al: Proton irradiation of malignant melanoma of the ciliary body. Br J Ophthalmol 1979; 63:135–139.
14 Damato B, et al: Proton beam radiotherapy of iris melanoma. Int J Radiat Oncol Biol Phys 2005;63: 109–115.
15 Damato B, Kacperek A, Chopra M, Campbell IR, Errington RD: Proton beam radiotherapy of choroidal melanoma: the Liverpool-Clatterbridge experience. Int J Radiat Oncol Biol Phys 2005;62:1405–1411.
16 Fuss M, Loredo LN, Blacharski PA, Grove RI, Slater JD: Proton radiation therapy for medium and large choroidal melanoma: preservation of the eye and its functionality. Int J Radiat Oncol Biol Phys 2001;49: 1053–1059.
17 Kacperek A: Proton therapy of eye tumours in the UK: a review of treatment at Clatterbridge. Appl Radiat Isot 2009;67:378–386.
18 Goyal S, Cohler A, Camporeale J, Narra V, Yue NJ: Intensity-modulated radiation therapy for orbital lymphoma. Radiat Med 2008;26:573–581.
19 Hein PA, Gladstone DJ, Bellerive MR, Hug EB: Importance of protocol target definition on the ability to spare normal tissue: an IMRT and 3D-CRT planning comparison for intraorbital tumors. Int J Radiat Oncol Biol Phys 2005;62:1540–1548.
20 Reisner ML, et al: Retinoblastoma – comparative analysis of external radiotherapy techniques, including an IMRT technique. Int J Radiat Oncol Biol Phys 2007;67:933–941.
21 Lightstone AW, et al: Cone beam CT (CBCT) evaluation of inter- and intra-fraction motion for patients undergoing brain radiotherapy immobilized using a commercial thermoplastic mask on a robotic couch. Technol Cancer Res Treat 2012;11:203–209.
22 Zumsteg Z, et al: Image guidance during head-and-neck cancer radiation therapy: analysis of alignment trends with in-room cone-beam computed tomography scans. Int J Radiat Oncol Biol Phys 2012;83: 712–719.

23 Dionisi F, et al: Set-up errors and planning target volume margins in head and neck cancer radiotherapy: a clinical study of image guidance with on-line cone-beam computed tomography. Int J Clin Oncol 2012. doi:10.1007/s10147-012-0395-7.
24 Mao W, et al: Initial application of a geometric QA tool for integrated MV and kV imaging systems on three image guided radiotherapy systems. Med Phys 2011;38:2335–2341.
25 Shin D, et al: Eye tracking and gating system for proton therapy of orbital tumors. Med Phys 2012;39: 4265.
26 McQuaid D, Webb S: IMRT delivery to a moving target by dynamic MLC tracking: delivery for targets moving in two dimensions in the beam's eye view. Phys Med Biol 2006;51:4819–4839.
27 Riboldi M, Orecchia R, Baroni G: Real-time tumour tracking in particle therapy: technological developments and future perspectives. Lancet Oncol 2012; 13:e383–e391.
28 Jaywant SM, Osei EK, Ladak S: Stereotactic radiotherapy in the treatment of ocular melanoma: a noninvasive eye fixation aid and tracking system. J Appl Clin Med Phys 2003;4:156–161.
29 Leksell L: The stereotaxic method and radiosurgery of the brain. Acta Chir Scand 1951;102:316–319.
30 Kang DW, Lee SC, Park YG, Chang JH: Long-term results of Gamma Knife surgery for uveal melanomas. J Neurosurg 2012;117(suppl):108–114.
31 Dinca EB, et al: Survival and complications following γ knife radiosurgery or enucleation for ocular melanoma: a 20-year experience. Acta Neurochir (Wien) 2012;154:605–610.
32 Rennie I, Forster D, Kemeny A, Walton L, Kunkler I: The use of single fraction Leksell stereotactic radiosurgery in the treatment of uveal melanoma. Acta Ophthalmol Scand 1996;74:558–562.
33 Kim CY, Lee SY: Orbital paraganglioma: gamma knife surgery as a therapeutic option. J Craniofac Surg 2012;23:1127–1128.
34 Kim YT, Kang SW, Lee J-I: Gamma knife radiosurgery for choroidal hemangioma. Int J Radiat Oncol Biol Phys 2011;81:1399–1404.
35 Sarici AM, Pazarli H: Gamma-knife-based stereotactic radiosurgery for medium- and large-sized posterior uveal melanoma. Graefes Arch Clin Exp Ophthalmol 2013;251:285–294.
36 Marchini G, et al: Gamma Knife stereotactic radiosurgery of ocular metastases: a case report. Stereotact Funct Neurosurg 1995;64(suppl 1):67–71.
37 Hayashi M, et al: Gamma Knife surgery for abducent nerve schwannoma. Report of 4 cases. J Neurosurg 2010;113(suppl):136–143.
38 Xu D, et al: Gamma Knife surgery in the management of orbital tumors. J Neurosurg 2010;113(suppl): 34–38.
39 Hungerford JL, et al: Side effects of photon and proton radiotherapy for ocular melanoma. Front Radiat Ther Oncol 1997;30:287–293.
40 Paganetti H, et al: Assessment of radiation-induced second cancer risks in proton therapy and IMRT for organs inside the primary radiation field. Phys Med Biol 2012;57:6047–6061.
41 Höcht S, et al: Proton or stereotactic photon irradiation for posterior uveal melanoma? Strahlenther Onkol 2005;181:783–788.
42 Toktas ZO, et al: Gamma knife stereotactic radiosurgery yields good long-term outcomes for low-volume uveal melanomas without intraocular complications. J Clin Neurosci 2010;17:441–445.
43 Furdova A, et al: One-day session LINAC-based stereotactic radiosurgery of posterior uveal melanoma. Eur J Ophthalmol 2012;22:226–235.
44 Furdova A, et al: No differences in outcome between radical surgical treatment (enucleation) and stereotactic radiosurgery in patients with posterior uveal melanoma. Neoplasma 2010;57:377–381.
45 Bianciotto C, Shields CL, Lally SE, Freire J, Shields JA: CyberKnife radiosurgery for the treatment of intraocular and periocular lymphoma. Arch Ophthalmol 2010;128:1561–1567.
46 Zehetmayer M, et al: Local tumor control and morbidity after one to three fractions of stereotactic external beam irradiation for uveal melanoma. Radiother Oncol 2000;55:135–144.
47 Zehetmayer M, et al: Fractionated stereotactic radiotherapy with linear accelerator for uveal melanoma – preliminary Vienna results. Strahlenther Onkol 1999;175(suppl 2):74–75.
48 Zorlu F, Selek U, Kiratli H: Initial results of fractionated CyberKnife radiosurgery for uveal melanoma. J Neuro-Oncol 2009;94:111–117.
49 Hirschbein MJ, Collins S, Jean WC, Chang SD, Adler JR: Treatment of intraorbital lesions using the Accuray CyberKnife system. Orbit 2008;27:97–105.
50 Weber DC, et al: Proton beam radiotherapy versus fractionated stereotactic radiotherapy for uveal melanomas: a comparative study. Int J Radiat Oncol Biol Phys 2005;63:373–384.
51 Al-Wassia R, et al: Stereotactic fractionated radiotherapy in the treatment of juxtapapillary choroidal melanoma: the McGill University experience. Int J Radiat Oncol Biol Phys 2011;81:e455–e462.
52 Raju MR: Proton radiobiology, radiosurgery and radiotherapy. Int J Radiat Biol 1995;67:237–259.
53 Koch NC, Newhauser WD: Development and verification of an analytical algorithm to predict absorbed dose distributions in ocular proton therapy using Monte Carlo simulations. Phys Med Biol 2010;55: 833–853.

54 Rethfeldt C, Fuchs H, Gardey KU: Dose distributions of a proton beam for eye tumor therapy: hybrid pencil-beam ray-tracing calculations. Med Phys 2006;33:782–791.
55 Koch N, et al: Monte Carlo calculations and measurements of absorbed dose per monitor unit for the treatment of uveal melanoma with proton therapy. Phys Med Biol 2008;53:1581–1594.
56 Baker CR, Quine TE, Brunt JNH, Kacperek A: Monte Carlo simulation and polymer gel dosimetry of 60 MeV clinical proton beams for the treatment of ocular tumours. Appl Radiat Isot 2009;67:402–405.
57 Salvadori RP, Rembado D, Serrato R: Proton-therapy, present status. Panminerva Med 1993;35:117–119.
58 Gragoudas ES: The Bragg peak of proton beams for treatment of uveal melanoma. Int Ophthalmol Clin 1980;20:123–133.
59 Jette D, Chen W: Creating a spread-out Bragg peak in proton beams. Phys Med Biol 2011;56:N131–N138.
60 Archambault L, et al: Verification of proton range, position, and intensity in IMPT with a 3D liquid scintillator detector system. Med Phys 2012;39:1239–1246.
61 Khan FM: The Physics of Radiation Therapy. Philadelphia, Lippincott Williams & Wilkins, 2010.
62 Schippers JM, Lomax AJ: Emerging technologies in proton therapy. Acta Oncol 2011;50:838–850.
63 Daftari IK, et al: Anterior segment sparing to reduce charged particle radiotherapy complications in uveal melanoma. Int J Radiat Oncol Biol Phys 1997;39:997–1010.
64 Castro JR, et al: Current status of clinical particle radiotherapy at Lawrence Berkeley Laboratory. Cancer 1980;46:633–641.
65 Grizzard WS, Torczynski E, Char DH: Helium ion charged-particle therapy for choroidal melanoma. Histopathologic findings in a successfully treated case. Arch Ophthalmol 1984;102:576–578.
66 Char DH, Kroll SM, Castro J: Long-term follow-up after uveal melanoma charged particle therapy. Trans Am Ophthalmol Soc 1997;95:171–187.
67 Orecchia R, et al: Particle beam therapy (hadrontherapy): basis for interest and clinical experience. Eur J Cancer 1998;34:459–468.
68 Saunders WM, et al: Precision, high dose radiotherapy: helium ion treatment of uveal melanoma. Int J Radiat Oncol Biol Phys 1985;11:227–233.

Roger Macklis, MD
Department of Radiation Oncology, Cleveland Clinic Foundation
9500 Euclid Avenue T-28
Cleveland, OH 44195 (USA)
E-Mail macklir@ccf.org

Singh AD, Pelayes DE, Seregard S, Macklis R (eds): Ophthalmic Radiation Therapy. Techniques and Applications.
Dev Ophthalmol. Basel, Karger, 2013, vol 52, pp 29–35 (DOI: 10.1159/000351053)

Brachytherapy

Gaurav Marwaha[a] · Roger Macklis[a] · Arun D. Singh[b] · Allan Wilkinson[a]

[a]Department of Radiation Oncology, Taussig Cancer Center and [b]Department of Ophthalmic Oncology, Cole Eye Institute, Cleveland Clinic Foundation, Cleveland, Ohio, USA

Abstract

Brachytherapy is the preferred radiation treatment modality for various intraocular tumors, most commonly, uveal melanoma. Radioactive sources are placed directly onto or around the tumor with the aid of episcleral plaques, whereby the employed sources exhibit an extremely sharp fall-off of dosage outside the few millimeters around the tumor. With such high focality, radiation dose to vision critical structures is minimized. Various sources have been used over the years, with iodine-125 being the most common. This chapter will highlight the history of brachytherapy for the treatment of intraocular tumors, current practice including isotopes and plaques utilized, as well as a comprehensive treatment planning and physics review.

Historical Perspective

'Brachy' therapy literally means 'short' therapy (in Greek), referring to the distance between the source of radiation and the treatment target. Its greatest therapeutic advantage is that its dose distribution follows an 'inverse square law', whereby exposure rate is equal to $1/r^2$ at a distance, r, from the source. In other words, dose delivered locally to a tumor can be extremely high while nearby normal tissues receive less dose. Brachytherapy can be delivered via three mechanisms: interstitial, intracavitary, and surface application. Radium, discovered in 1898, was the first isotope used in brachytherapy [1]. Such radioisotopes decay into more stable forms, and in turn, release ionizing radiation that has the capacity to inflict double strand DNA breakage, and ultimately cell death.

Brachytherapy for ocular tumors was pioneered in 1930, when Foster Moore began using interstitial therapy for uveal melanoma, using seeds of radon as his sour-

Table 1. Isotopes commonly utilized in brachytherapy, with their respective properties

Radionuclide	Decay mode	Energy	Half-life
Pd-103	electron capture	21 keV	17 days
I-125	electron capture	28 keV	60.2 days
Cs-131	electron capture	30.4 KeV	9.7 days
Ru-106	beta minus	3.54 MeV	373.59 days
Sr-90	beta minus	970 keV	28 years

ce [2]. In the 1940s, Stallard began to use seeds of cobalt-60 for the treatment of rhabdomyosarcoma. These seeds were shielded with heavy metal (silver and gold) plaques. Cobalt-60, however, had limitations with dose distribution customization. Additionally, the toxicities for radon and cobalt-60 proved to be excessive, leading to the introduction of other isotopes, specifically ^{125}I, ^{103}Pd, ^{106}Ru, ^{131}Cs, and ^{90}Sr. Table 1 highlights the properties of the most commonly utilized brachytherapy sources today.

Isotopes

These modern radioisotopes allow easy integration of sufficient shielding within the plaque, which is imperative, as it mitigates radiation dosage to other parts of the eye, and absorbs 99% of the radiation, allowing for safety of healthcare workers and patient visitors [2]. Hence, most plaques are made of gold or silver. The latter is used for ^{106}Ru for technical reasons.

Nowadays ^{125}I is the most commonly utilized photon radiation source for eye plaque brachytherapy. Its advantages, in particular, include a half-life conducive for storage, and low photon energy, requiring less shielding [1]. The isotope decays via electron capture to ^{125}Te, which, in an excited state, immediately decays to its ground state while emitting a 35.5 keV photon [1]. Additionally, therapeutic K-X rays, ranging from 27 to 31 keV, are produced. The iodine seeds are encapsulated in 0.05 mm titanium tubes welded at each end. The titanium aids in absorbing any electrons or L-x-rays with small, insignificant energies. The end welds create an anisotropic dose distribution [1]. This phenomenon is depicted in figure 1.

As a beta emitter, ^{106}Ru is particularly adequate to treat circumscribed lesions like ophthalmic tumors. ^{106}Ru decays via low energy β^- emission with a half-life of 373.6 days. The therapeutic dose, however, arises from the subsequent β^- decay of the daughter nuclide ^{106}Rh with a maximum energy of 3.54 MeV. The steep dose fall-off is for β-radiation.

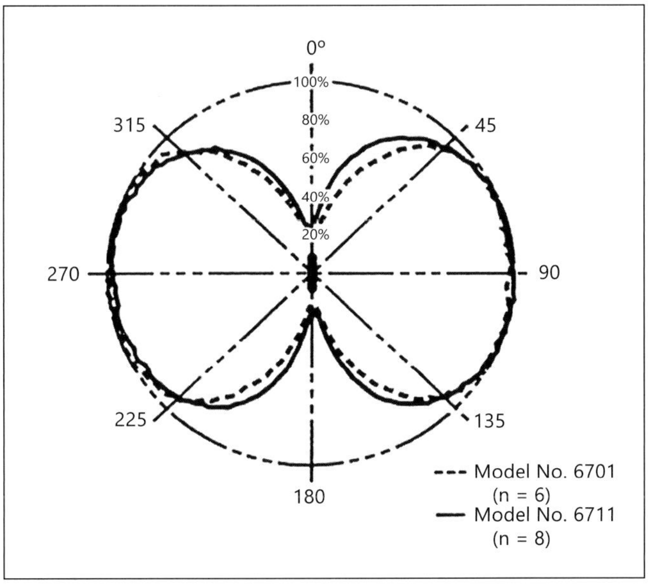

Fig. 1. Anisotropic fluence observed with ^{125}I seeds.

Radiation Plaques

All plaques are episcleral, emitting the therapeutic radiation only on the concave side. To achieve this, either radiation sources (e.g. ^{125}I seeds) are glued/molded onto an inactive carrier or a radioactive layer is integrated into the plaque itself, as it is the case in Ru-106 eye applicators. Two or more eyelets allow the plaque to be sutured to the scleral surface.

The most commonly used plaque in the USA is the Collaborative Ocular Melanoma Study (COMS) plaque, which comes in a range of sizes (10–20 mm) and may be notched for proximity to the optic nerve. The COMS plaques can be individually loaded with up to 24 seeds. A silastic insert with a fixed matrix of slots allows for reproducible seed positioning which is mandatory for radiation treatment planning. Seeds and the gold shells can be reused (fig. 2).

In Europe, ^{106}Ru applicators were introduced in the 1960s by Lommatzsch and remain in use today. Unlike the COMS plaques, ^{106}Ru applicators do not require any assembly. The radioactive material is electrodeposited on a thin silver foil mounted between a 0.7-mm silver backing and a 0.1-mm silver window. This design leads to a thin (1-mm) and therefore notably handy applicator. The plaques are reusable for 1 year. Circular plaques with different diameters from 11 to 25 mm and also several notched geometries are available (fig. 3).

Change of Paradigm

The treatment of tumors like uveal melanoma was historically surgical, namely enucleation, and it wasn't until a series of studies towards the end of the 20th century that the pendulum swung towards brachytherapy. A large retrospective study from

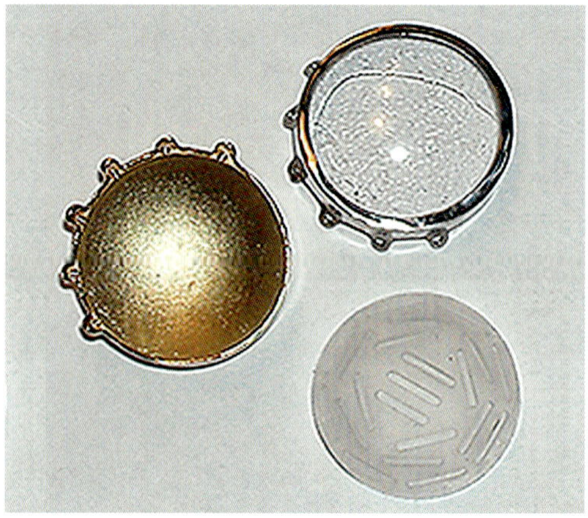

Fig. 2. COMS ^{125}I eye plaque. Note that the COMS plaque includes a silastic insert.

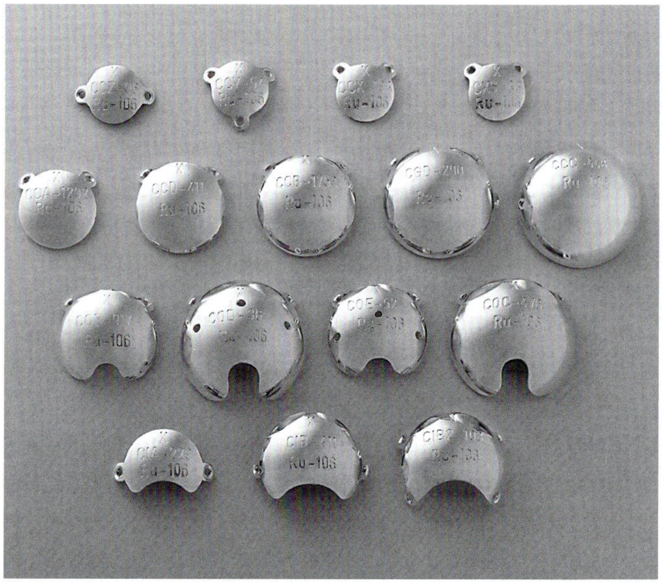

Fig. 3. ^{106}Ru eye plaque. Circular and notched plaques with different diameters from 11 to 25 mm are available. Courtesy of Eckert & Ziegler BEBIG, Berlin, Germany.

the Manhattan Eye, Ear and Throat Hospital in the 1980s revealed similar oncologic outcomes between cobalt plaques and enucleation for the management of uveal melanoma [3]. These findings prompted the COMS, a set of clinical trials in the 1980s–1990s, where medium-sized (defined as tumor height 2.5–10 mm and diameter ≤16 mm) tumors were randomized to ^{125}I seeds or enucleation [4]. Brachytherapy was conducted using an episcleral plaque with a 2–3 mm margin around the base of the tumor, with a dose of 85 Gy prescribed to 5 mm from the inner surface of the sclera for smaller tumors and prescribed to the apex for tumors >5 mm. The use of a silastic carrier with slots for the sources gave reproducibility to the im-

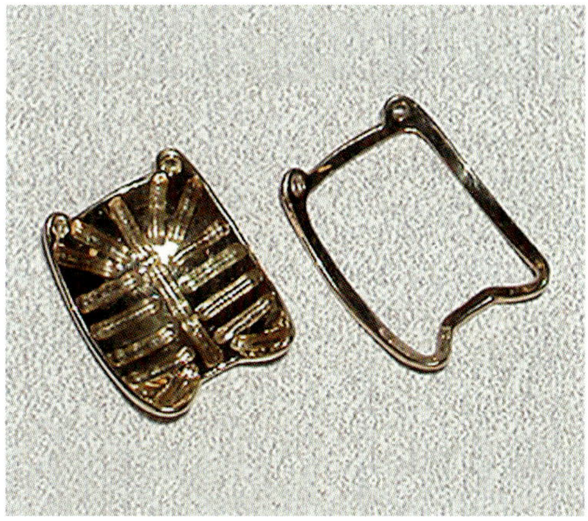

Fig. 4. EP917 ^{125}I eye plaque. Note slimmer design and absence of silastic insert.

plants. The dosimetry was made purposely simple. That is, full scatter in a water medium and a point source with an isotropic fluence pattern were assumed. COMS data revealed that brachytherapy with ^{125}I seeds offered equivalent overall (OS) and metastasis-free survival (DMFS) compared to enucleation at 12 years: OS of 57 versus 59% and DMFS of 21 versus 17%, respectively [4]. This randomized trial set the precedent for the modern era of accepting plaque brachytherapy as the less toxic treatment standard.

Current Practice and Recent Developments

The American Brachytherapy Society issued recommendations in 2003 for plaque therapy that specified a minimum ^{125}I apical dose of 85 Gy at a dose rate of 0.6–1.05 Gy/h using TG43. This assumes approximation of the point source, no anisotropy corrections, no backscatter from shielding, and use of a silastic insert [5]. ^{125}I is preferred given its low energy and usage in the COMS trials. That was followed in the same year by a reanalysis of COMS dosimetry [6] that showed significant reductions in doses to structures of interest, including tumor apex (>10%), when anisotropy, line source approximation, and silastic and gold shield attenuation were taken into account. A more recent set of recommendations for COMS plaque use comes from the report of Task Group 129 of the AAPM and ABS [7]. It recommends the use of line-source approximation in homogeneous water medium, and the two-dimensional AAPM TG-43U1 formalism and source parameters. This also applies to the use of ^{103}Pd, which is similar to ^{125}I, in that the photon energies are lower. Tables providing estimates of the central axis doses calculated using heterogeneity corrections for all sizes of COMS plaques and one seed model for each of the two radionuclides are given. These dose calculations were based on Monte Carol studies by Thomson et al. [8]. There are currently two treatment planning systems available

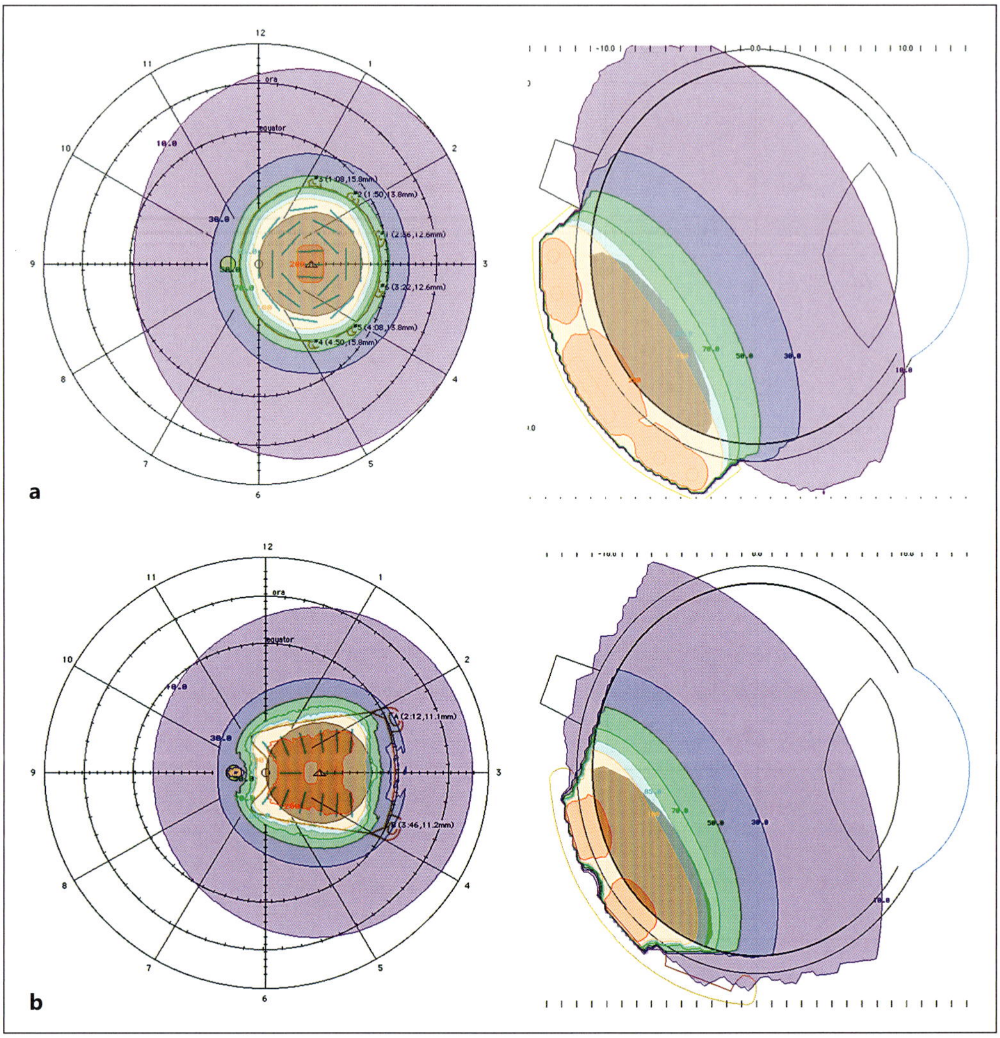

Fig. 5. Retinal (left) and volumetric prescription isodose (right) diagrams of COMS (**a**) versus EP917 (**b**) plaque for the same tumor. Note the similar tumor coverage between the two plaques, despite less nontumoral dose with the EP917 plaque.

for making such calculations (Brachydose and Plaque Simulator). Both yield very similar dose estimates on axis [9].

^{106}Ru, the preferred isotope in Europe, offers an even faster dose fall-off than ^{125}I and therefore an inherent advantage, which can aid in sparing of vision critical structures. As a matter of fact, this source may give very high doses to sclera when treating larger lesions, hence it is best utilized in management of smaller melanomas [10]. It allows to reliably treat tumors up to 5.4 mm in height. In a study with 458 patients, Damato [11, 12] achieved actuarial rates of tumor recurrence of 1, 2 and 3% at 2, 5 and 7 years, respectively.

Treatment toxicity is primarily related to vision loss from retinopathy and optic neuropathy. The major modifiable risk factor for these toxicities is total radiation dose to the macula and optic disc [6]. One of the ways to accomplish this is to improve on standard COMS plaque design. More modern, slimmer plaque designs (Eye Physics) may take advantage of collimation to reduce toxicity (fig. 4). Such plaques do not need a silastic carrier, as seeds are glued into the grooves of the gold casing. This allows for dose homogeneity within the tumor to be improved while minimizing adjacent dose scatter to critical structures. While the dosimetry is conformal and promising with this approach (fig. 5), clinical benefit is yet to be proven [6].

References

1 Khan FM: Brachytherapy; in Khan FM (ed): The Physics of Radiation Therapy, ed 3. Philadelphia, Lippincott Williams & Wilkins, 2003, pp 357–400.

2 Seregard S, Damato B, Fleming P: Uveal malignant melanoma: management options – brachytherapy; in Singh AD, Damato BE, Pe'er J, Murphree AL, Perry JD (eds): Clinical Ophthalmic Oncology, ed 1. Philadelphia, Saunders Elsevier, 2007, pp 241–247.

3 Adams KS, et al: Cobalt plaque versus enucleation for uveal melanoma: comparison of survival rates. Br J Ophthalmol 1988;72:494–497.

4 Collaborative Ocular Melanoma Study Group: The COMS randomized trial of iodine 125 brachytherapy for choroidal melanoma. V. Twelve-year mortality rates and prognostic factors: COMS report No. 28. Arch Ophthalmol 2006;124:1684–1693.

5 Nag S, et al: The American Brachytherapy Society recommendations for brachytherapy of uveal melanomas. Int J Radiat Oncol Biol Phys 2003;56:544–555.

6 Krintz AL, et al: A reanalysis of the collaborative ocular melanoma study medium tumor trial eye plaque dosimetry. Int J Radiat Oncol Biol Phys 2003;56: 889–898.

7 Chiu-Tsao ST, et al: Dosimetry of 125I and 103Pd COMS eye plaques for intraocular tumors: report of Task Group 129 by the AAPM and ABS. Med Phys 2012;39:6161–6184.

8 Thomson RM, et al: Monte Carlo dosimetry for ^{125}I and ^{103}Pd eye plaque brachytherapy. Med Phys 2008; 35:5530–5543.

9 Marwaha G, Wilkinson A, Bena J, Macklis R, Singh A: Dosimetric benefit of a new ophthalmic radiation plaque. Int J Radiat Oncol Biol Phys 2012;84:1226–1230.

10 Wilkinson DA: Dosimetric comparison of Ru-106 and I-125 plaques for treatment of shallow (≤5 mm) choroidal melanoma lesions. Br J Radiol 2008;81: 784–789.

11 Damato B: Local tumor control after Ru-106 Brachytherapy of choroidal melanoma. Int J Radiat Oncol Biol Phys 2005;63:385–391.

12 Damato B: Visual acuity after Ru-106 brachytherapy of choroidal melanomas. Int J Radiat Oncol Biol Phys 2005;63:392–400.

Allan Wilkinson, PhD
Department of Radiation Oncology
Cleveland Clinic Foundation, Desk T-28
9500 Euclid Avenue, Cleveland, OH 44195 (USA)
E-Mail wilkina@ccf.org

Singh AD, Pelayes DE, Seregard S, Macklis R (eds): Ophthalmic Radiation Therapy. Techniques and Applications.
Dev Ophthalmol. Basel, Karger, 2013, vol 52, pp 36–57 (DOI: 10.1159/000351055)

Radiation Therapy: Uveal Tumors

Stefan Seregard[a] · David E. Pelayes[b] · Arun D. Singh[c]

[a]St Eriks Eye Hospital, Karolinska Institutet, Stockholm, Sweden; [b]Department of Ophthalmology, Maimonides University, Buenos Aires, Argentina; [c]Department of Ophthalmic Oncology, Cole Eye Institute, Cleveland Clinic Foundation, Cleveland, Ohio, USA

Abstract

Among primary uveal tumors, uveal melanoma is the most frequently occurring malignant neoplasm, albeit much less common than skin melanoma and indeed most other cancers. Traditionally, uveal melanoma was treated by enucleation of the globe, but is now increasingly been managed by an eye-preserving option, which saves vision without compromising the life of patients. More than 90% of eyes now preserved have some form of radiotherapy; most often episcleral brachytherapy that is easily accessible at many ophthalmic centers. Conversely, teletherapy in the form of charged particle irradiation, stereotactic radiotherapy or radiosurgery is only available at a comparatively small number of centers. Radiotherapy for uveal melanoma causes significant side effects and complications, but the vast majority of patients can keep their eye with some remaining function. This is of significant benefit to the quality of life for many patients. The side effects of radiotherapy are intimately related to the size of the irradiated tumor, hence early detection and identification of tumors that need to be treated is critical to improve the functional outcome. Experience gained from treating uveal melanoma has been expanded to treat benign uveal tumors such as choroidal hemangioma and other malignant tumors such as uveal lymphoma and uveal metastasis.

Uveal Melanoma

Uveal melanoma arises from the melanocytes of the uveal tract, i.e. from the neural crest derived nonepithelial, pigment-containing cells of the choroid, ciliary body and iris stroma. In most cases no precursor lesion can be identified, but it is widely assumed that most lesions arise from uveal nevi which transform into melanoma. Individuals with syndromes like oculo(dermal) melanocytosis are at an increased risk to develop uveal melanoma [1, 2], but the vast majority of uveal melanoma occur in patients with no apparent predisposing condition. Moreover, most cases occur in a sporadic setting and familial uveal melanoma is distinctly uncommon, although an increasing number of families with germline BAP-1 mutations and familial uveal melanoma are now being reported [3, 4]. Intriguing new evidence also suggest that GNAQ and GNA11 mutations occur early in tumorigenesis, but that BAP1 mutations are required for a metastatic phenotype [5]. Interestingly, the incidence of uveal melanoma is largely stable in many countries and does not parallel the rapid increase seen in cutaneous melanoma [6, 7]. Although, there are a few reports of uveal melanoma being more frequent in welders, occupational exposure to ultraviolet radiation has not been associated with uveal melanoma [8]. This strongly suggests that ultraviolet radiation, believed to cause much of cutaneous melanoma, is much less, if at all, implicated in uveal melanoma pathogenesis. Unlike cutaneous melanoma, mutations in the BRAF and BRAS genes are uncommon events in uveal melanoma [9–11]. Taken together, this suggests that the molecular mechanisms operating in uveal melanoma are different from those of cutaneous melanoma [12].

Diagnosis

Typically, a trained ophthalmologist can make the diagnosis by clinical appearance assisted by noninvasive techniques in 95% of the cases. Uveal melanoma is almost unique among cancers in that the clinical diagnosis often is not verified by cytological or histopathological examination. For tumors large enough to warrant enucleation, the clinical diagnosis is highly accurate at 99.7% [13]. For smaller tumors or clinically atypical tumors, diagnostic uncertainty can be resolved by any of a range of biopsy techniques [14]. Although symptoms like progressive visual filed loss and blurred vision are not specific for uveal melanoma, they usually warrant prompt ophthalmological examination. Still diagnostic delay and delays in referral to a dedicated ocular oncology center remains a concern [15]. Small melanocytic lesions are sometimes observed for growth before treatment is initiated, in particular when treatment is likely to be associated with significant visual loss. Features in indeterminate melanocytic lesions of the choroid like thickness greater than 2 mm, subretinal fluid, orange pigment, clinical symptoms, location within 3 mm of the optic disc, acoustic hollowness by ultrasonography and absence of halo are associated with increased risk for growth [16].

Management of Primary Disease

In the United States, there has been a dramatic shift towards the use of eye-preserving options for uveal melanoma. During 1973–1974, nearly all patients with uveal melanoma (98.3%) had surgery, almost always enucleation of the eye, but in 2004–2006

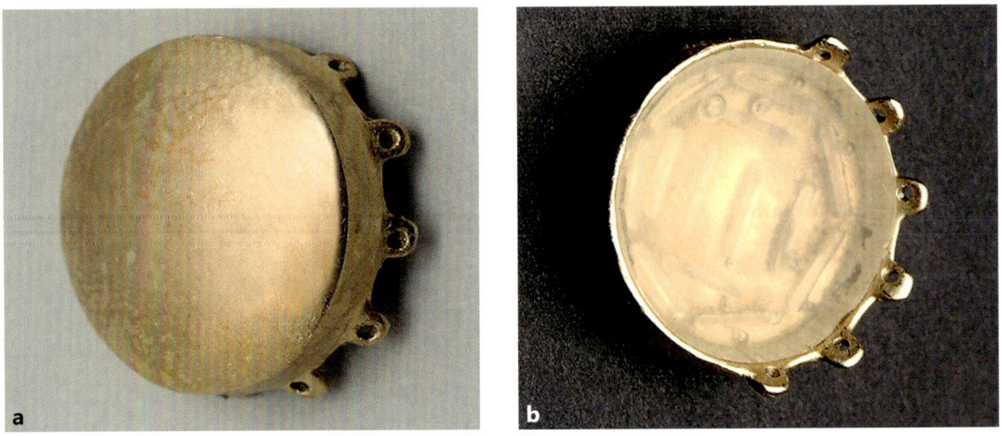

Fig. 1. Concave surface of COMS iodine-125 plaque (**a**). Note the iodine-125 seeds loaded in the gold disc. The convex surface is smooth (**b**).

only 28.3% of patients with uveal melanoma had surgery as the first option. During the same period of time, radiotherapy, largely episcleral brachytherapy, became much more common increasing dramatically as the first line of treatment from 1.8 to 62.5% of patients with uveal melanoma [7]. This change in strategy has been stimulated by evidence indicating that survival is not compromised for patients with medium-sized tumors have primary radiotherapy rather than enucleation and by the introduction of standardized plaques for episcleral brachytherapy as a result of the Collaborative Ocular Melanoma Study (COMS) [17].

However, the treatment is not standardized and patients with similarly sized tumors may receive different treatment depending on where they are managed and on the patient's preference. Enucleation is a reasonable option for many large tumors and tumors adjacent to the optic disc where poor visual outcome is expected [18]. Surgery is performed under general anesthesia and typically includes an orbital implant.

A range of radionuclides with different characteristics are available, iodine 125 has been popularized by the COMS in North America (fig. 1) but ruthenium 106 is more widely used in Europe (fig. 2) [19]. Episcleral brachytherapy may be performed in local anestehesia, but many surgeons prefer general anestehesia. The radioactive source is sutured to the episcleral surface overlying the tumor, typically including a 2-mm safety margin (fig. 2) [see chapter 'Brachytherapy' by Marwaha et al., this vol.]. Tissue penetration is greater for iodine and centers with access to both radionuclides often use ruthenium for small and medium-sized tumors and iodine for larger tumors (fig. 3) [17, 19–21].

A juxtapapillary choroidal melanoma is difficult to treat with episcleral brachytherapy and may be managed with proton beam radiotherapy and in some centers this technique is the first option for most uveal melanoma [22; see chapter 'Teletherapy:

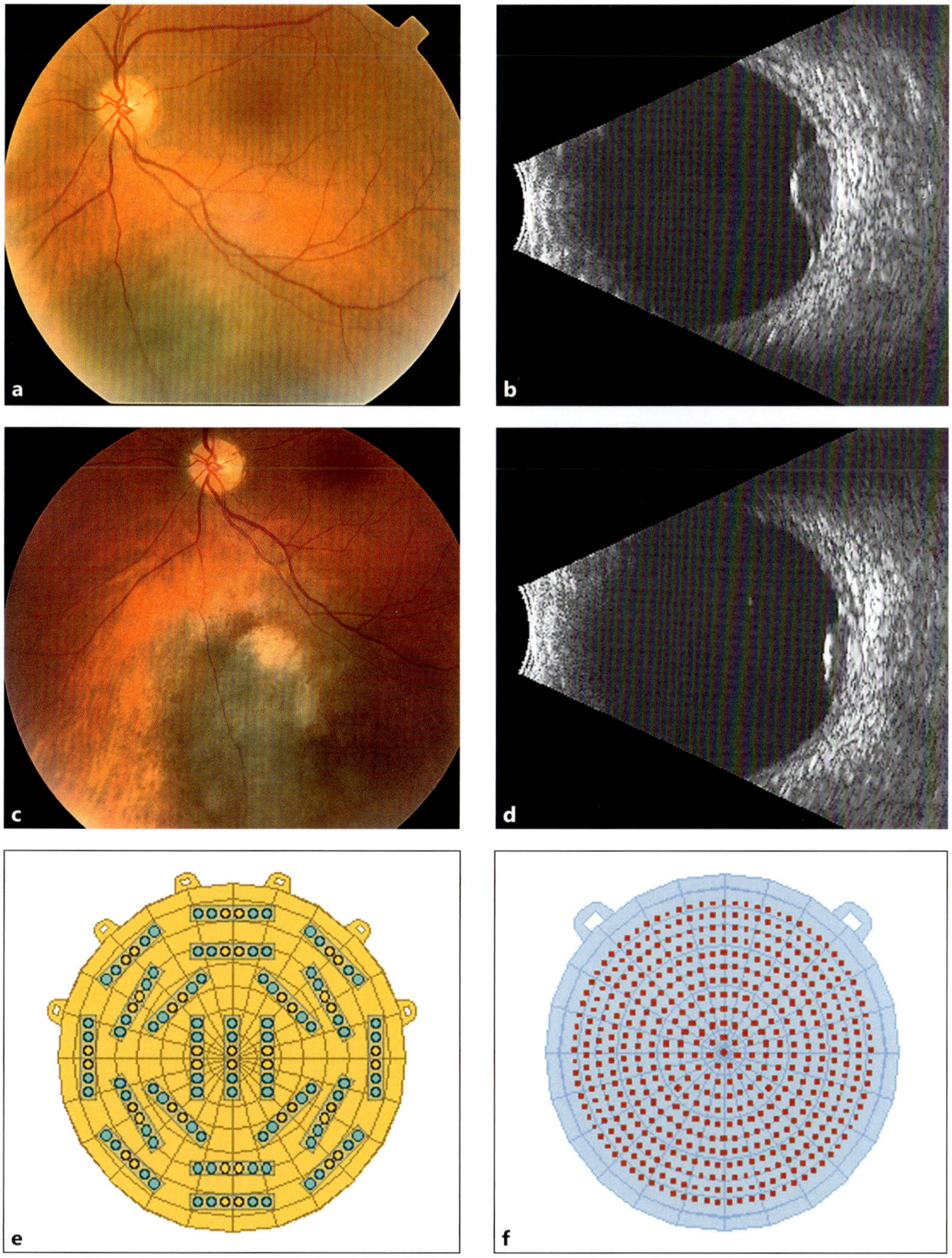

Fig. 2. **a** Fundus photograph showing a dome shaped pigmented choroidal melanoma with indistinct margins in the inferior quadrant OS. **b** The lesion had low internal reflectivity with absence of extrascleral extension). **c** Six months later, the tumor showed evidence of regression and complete resolution of exudative retinal detachment any radiation complications. **d** Tumor shrinkage is obvious on the B-scan ultrasonography. Schematic representation of iodine-125 plaque (**e**) and ruthenium-106 plaque (**f**).

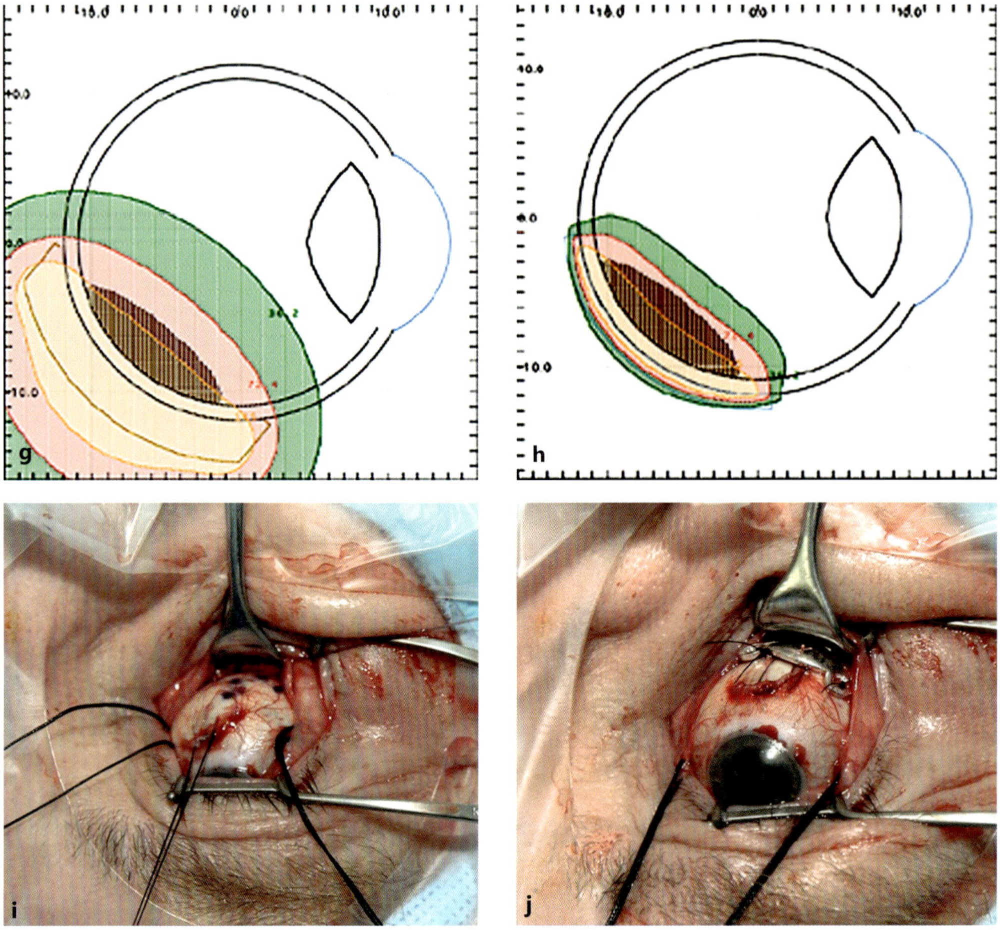

Fig. 2. Dose distribution curves with iodine-125 plaque (**g**) and ruthenium-106 plaque (**h**). Because of limited penetration of beta radiation of ruthenium 106 as compared with gamma radiation of iodine-125, the radiation distribution is limited to the immediate vicinity of the ruthenium-106 plaque. The tumor outline is marked on the sclera (**i**) and ruthenium-106 plaque sutured in place (**j**).

Advanced Techniques' by Stockham et al., this vol.]. To avoid significant side effects from radiation, large tumors may be fragmented and removed by a vitreous cutter (endoresection) a few weeks after radiotherapy [23]. Primary endoresection without the use of previous radiotherapy is highly controversial. Large tumors may also sometimes also be managed by transscleral local resection (exoresection) [23]. Alternative techniques used at some centers to treat uveal melanoma include fractionated stereotactic radiotherapy and single-fraction radiosurgery [24; see chapter 'Teletherapy: Advanced Techniques' by Stockham et al., this vol.]. Primary transpupillary thermotherapy is now rarely used as the sole therapy because of an increased risk for local recurrence and is now typically combined with brachytherapy [25].

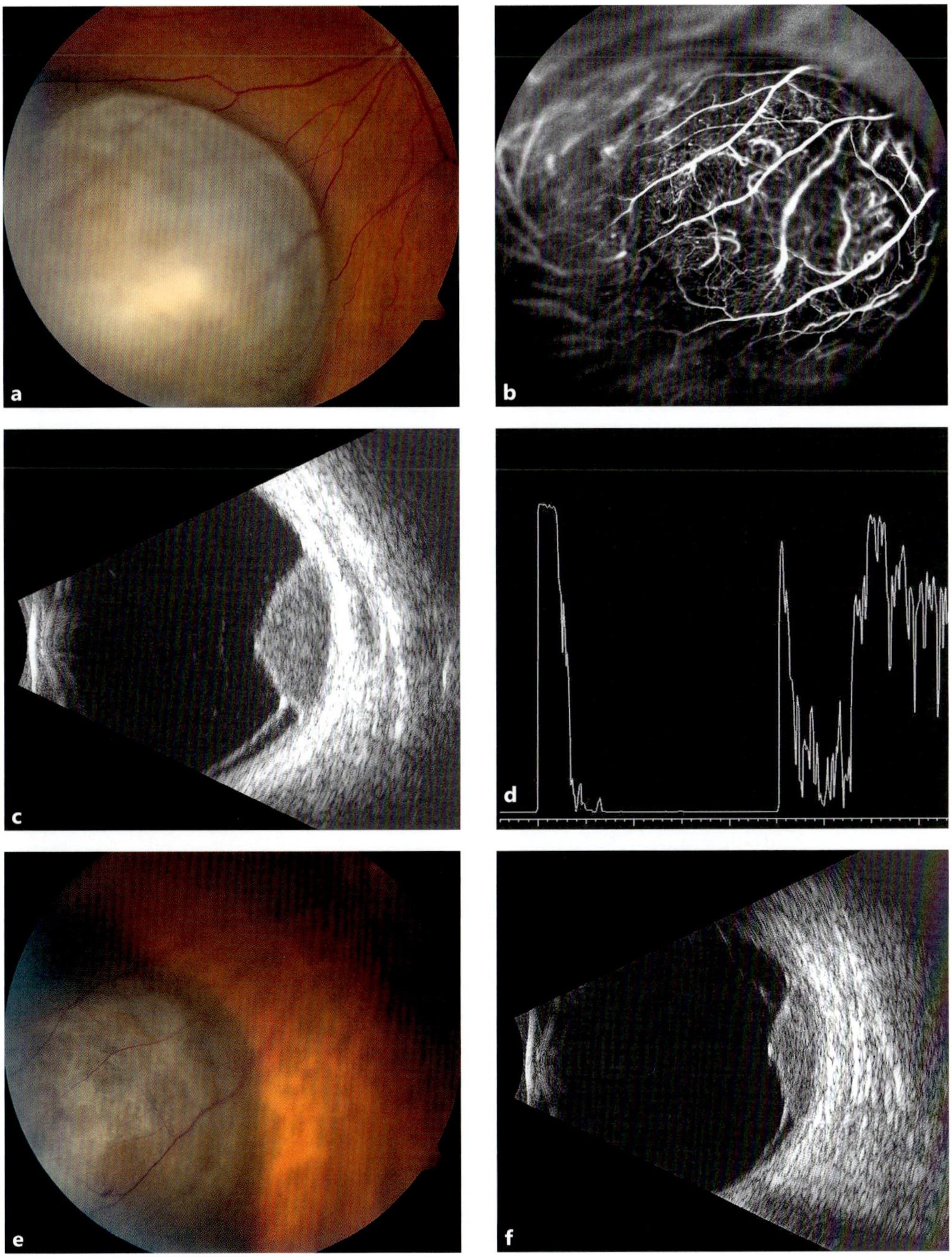

Fig. 3. Choroidal melanoma pretreatment fundus appearance (**a**), intrinsic vasculature on indocyanine angiogram (**b**), dome-shaped appearance on B scan ultrasonography (**c**) and low internal reflectivity on A scan ultrasonography (**d**) are characteristic features that support the clinical diagnosis. Three months after brachytherapy, note tumor shrinkage on ophthalmoscopic appearance (**e**) and B scan ultrasonography (**f**).

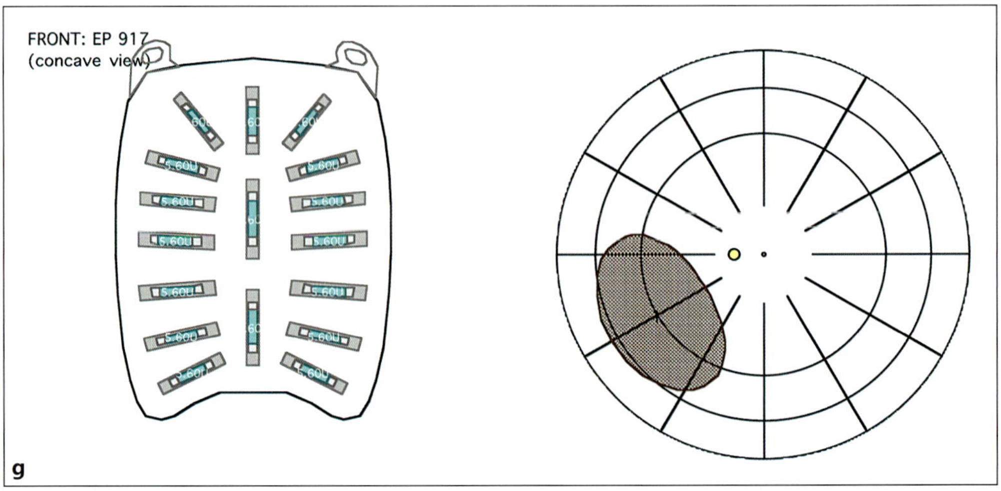

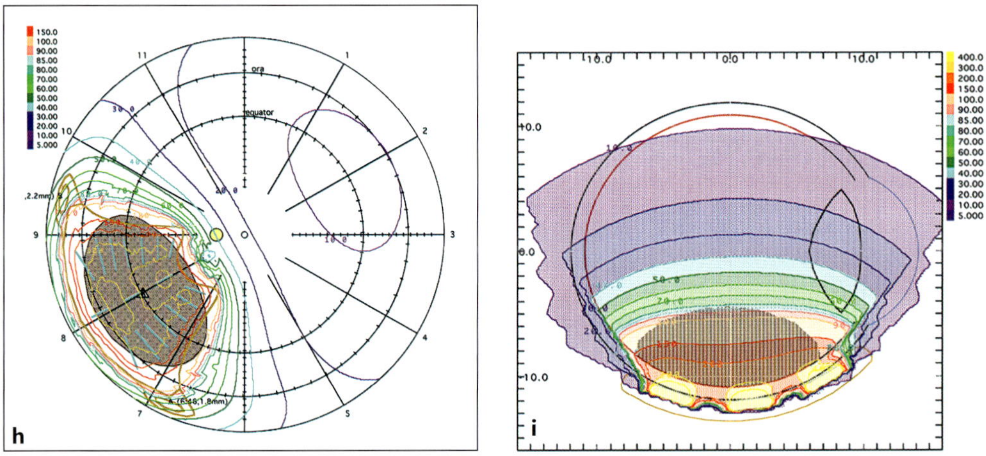

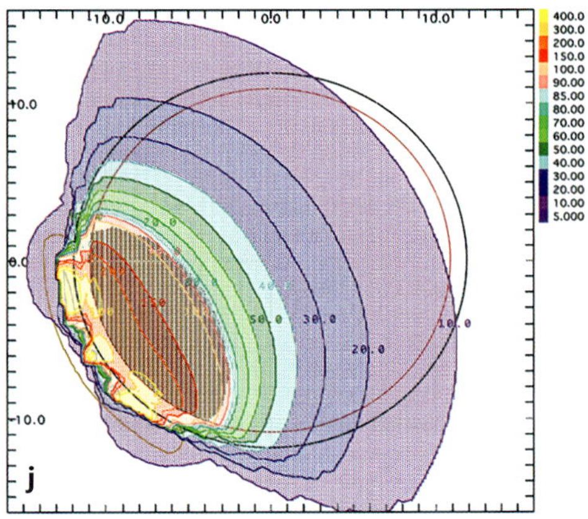

Fig. 3. Schematic representation of iodine-125 plaque (Eye Physics 917 design) and display of retinal diagram (**g**). Plaque simulator treatment plan with a prescribed dose of 83 Gy to the tumor apex (7.5 mm) (**h**), isodose plots (**i**, meridional view and **j**, equatorial view).

Follow-Up

Patients treated with an eye-preserving option are usually monitored periodically by an ophthalmologist for life. This includes comparison with standardized pretreatment fundus photographs and often ultrasonography. Patients with extrascleral growth found at or after enucleation may need periodic imaging of the orbit to exclude a local orbital recurrence. Uveal melanoma preferentially disseminates to the liver and systemic monitoring is typically focused to this site. Many centers offer liver imaging at periodic intervals after diagnosis [26]. Periodic monitoring of liver function tests is sometimes added, but sensitivity of serum liver enzymes to detect metastatic disease is low [27, 28].

Management of Systemic Disease

Traditionally, patients with systemic uveal melanoma often received treatment similar to patients with systemic cutaneous melanoma, but therapy is now more specific. Current strategies to manage systemic uveal melanoma include partial hepatectomy, radiofrequency ablation, elective internal radiotherapy, ipilimumab immunotherapy, liver chemoembolization, intrahepatic arterial chemotherapy and systemic chemotherapy [26]. Results from some of these therapies suggest that a subset of patients may have prolonged survival, although none of the strategies have efficacy proven in a randomized clinical trial.

Quality of Life

The diagnosis of ocular cancer generates significant anxiety and depression in patients [29, 30]. Symptoms like fatigue and insomnia are prevalent [29]. There is some data to suggest that anxiety diminishes faster after diagnosis in patients with enucleation than in patients with brachytherapy [30]. Visual function is initially better in patients with brachytherapy, but this difference is reduced with time as radiation related side effects emerge [30]. Differences between individuals may be significant.

Prognosis

Although significant progress has been made in the management of the primary uveal melanoma, prognosis for life has largely remained unchanged [31]. Notably, the mortality rate is higher than for patients with cutaneous melanoma and nearly half of patients with uveal melanoma will die with metastatic disease [32]. Most of these will die during the first 5 years after diagnosis [33], but some patients develop systemic disease several decades after diagnosis [34]. It is widely assumed that tumors spread when quite small, usually several years before diagnosis, and that metastases then remain unnoticed in the liver for many years [35, 36]. When metastatic disease becomes clinically evident, the median survival is less than 6 months [32]. Large tumors, anteriorly located tumors, tumors with specific extracellular matrix patterns and tumors containing epithelioid cells, cells with large nucleoli or a large proportion of cycling tumor cells carry a worse prognosis [36–38]. Moreover, tumors with chromosomal aberrations like monosomy 3 and gain of chromosome 8q are associated with poor survival [39, 40]. Recently, gene expression profiling has identified a subgroup of uveal melanoma associated with an extremely high mortality rate [41].

Circumscribed Choroidal Hemangioma

Benign, rare intraocular tumors, when circumscribed occur sporadically without any associated local or systemic anomalies [42, 43]. Circumscribed choroidal hemangioma is usually diagnosed between the second and fourth decades of life either as an incidental finding or due to visual symptoms such as reduced vision, metamorphopsia, photopsia or visual field defect.

Diagnosis

Ophthalmoscopically, it appears as an orange colored choroidal mass with indistinct margins located in the posterior pole and not thicker than 6 mm [43, 44]. A circumscribed choroidal hemangioma can be misdiagnosed as an amelanotic choroidal lesion such as an amelanotic choroidal malignant melanoma, choroidal metastasis, posterior scleritis, choroidal granuloma, choroidal osteoma, lymphoma or atypical central serous retinopathy. Ultrasonographic findings of high internal reflectivity and angiographic evidence of very early hyperfluorescence strongly support a diagnosis of cricumscribed choroidal hemangioma. On magenetic resonance imaging, choroidal hemangioma appears hyperintense to vitreous on T1-weighted MR images and isointense to vitreous on T2-weighted images with marked enhancement after gadolinium injection. This is in contrast, to hypointense appearance of choroidal melanoma in T2-weighted images [45].

Management of Primary Disease

The decision to treat is based upon the extent of symptoms, loss of vision, and the potential for visual recovery. The aim of treatment is to induce sufficient tumor atrophy with resolution of subretinal fluid and tumor-induced foveal distortion without de-

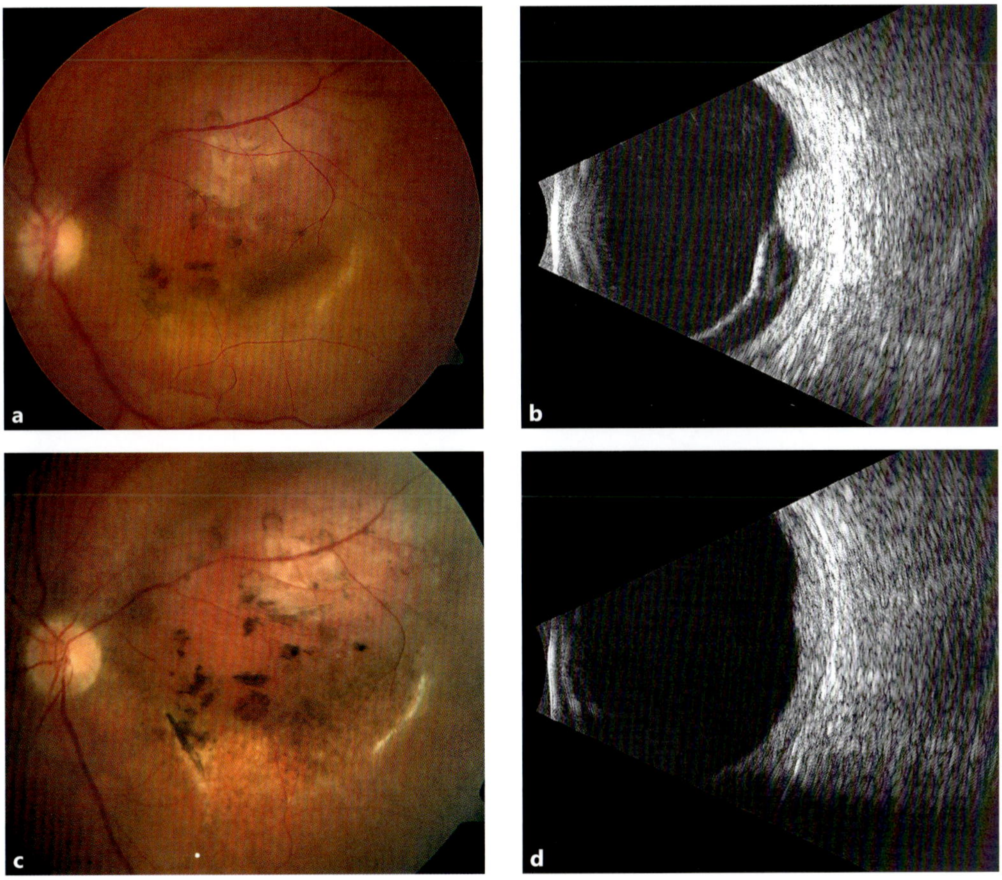

Fig. 4. Choroidal hemangioma treated with plaque radiation therapy. **a** Pretreatment fundus appearance with chronic exudative retinal detachment. **b** Ultrasonography appearance with thickness of 4.3 mm. Three months following treatment with iodine-125 plaque that delivered 33 Gy to the tumor apex over 44.5 h, note resolution of exudative retinal detachment (**c**) and regression of hemangioma (**d**, 2.6 mm height).

stroying the function of the overlying retina. Some asymptomatic cases can be observed. In cases where treatment is deemed necessary several options exist. Laser photocoagulation [42], cryotherapy, transpupillary thermotherapy [46], and radiotherapy have been reported to be efficacious for the treatment of circumscribed choroidal hemangioma. Photodynamic therapy with verteporfin (Visudyne™, Novartis Ophthalmics, Basel, Switzerland) is the treatment of choice [47–49].

In presence of extensive bullous retinal detachments or when other modalities of treatment have failed, radiation treatment for a circumscribed choroidal hemangioma can be delivered in several forms. In addition to lens-sparing external beam radiotherapy [50], stereotactic radiotherapy [51], plaque radiotherapy (cobalt-60, iodine-125, palladium-103) [52, 53], and proton beam radiotherapy has been used

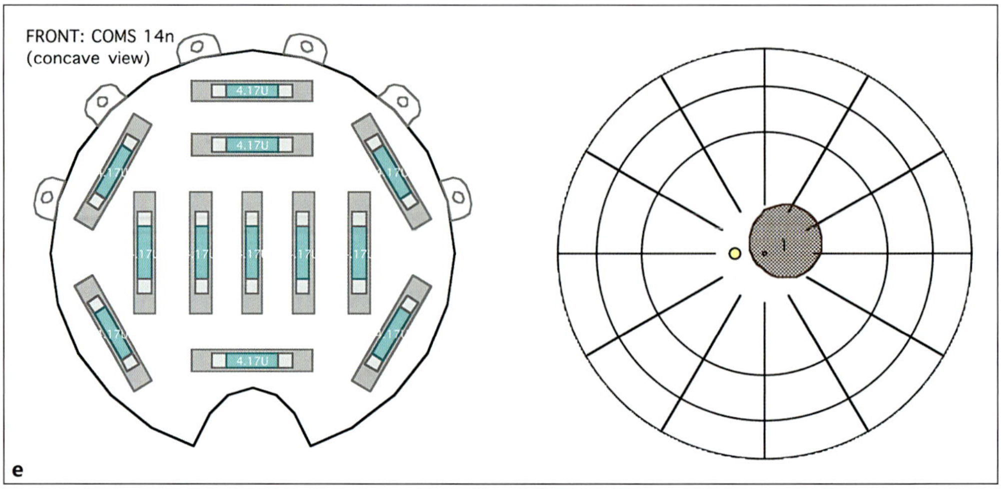

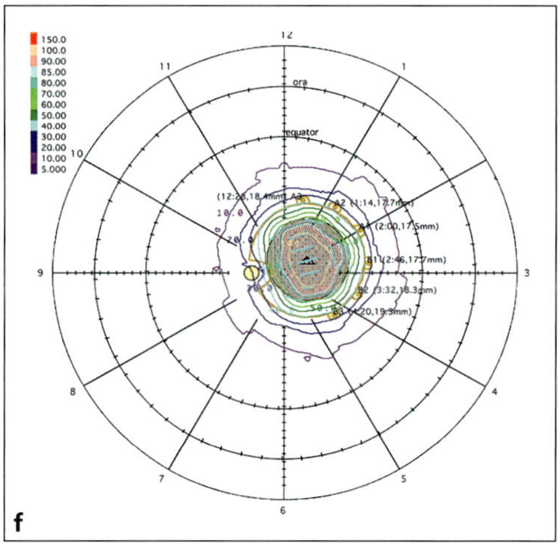

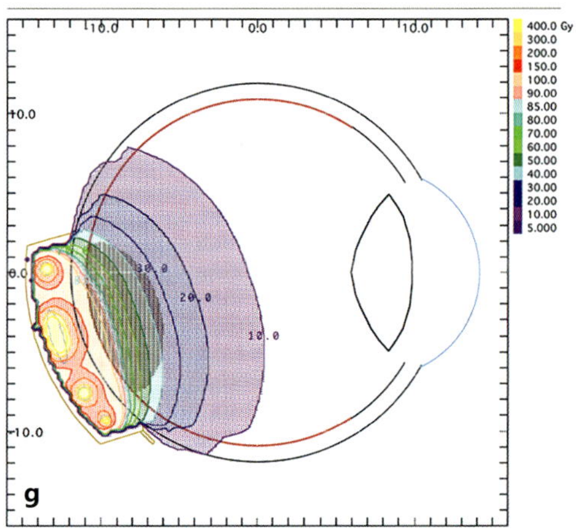

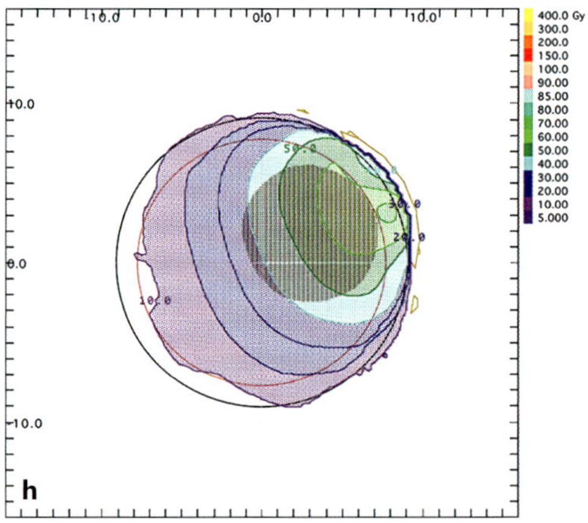

Fig. 4. Choroidal hemangioma treated with plaque radiation therapy. Plaque simulator treatment plan using 14-mm COMS notched plaque (**e**), display of retinal diagram with a prescribed dose of 33 Gy to the tumor apex (4.5 mm) (**f**), and isodose plots (**g**, meridional view and **h**, equatorial view).

(fig. 4) [54, 55]. In general, the total dosage used is about 20 Gy given in 10 fractions for external beam radiotherapy, 25–50 Gy for plaque radiotherapy, and 16.4–20.0 Gy in 4 fractions for proton beam radiotherapy. Stereotactic techniques, because of greater precision may be superior to other methods of radiation [51]. The technique of gamma knife radiosurgery has the advantage of delivering total radiation dose in a single session [56].

Prognosis

Resolution of exudative retinal detachment, tumor regression, and an improvement of vision in the majority of cases treated by radiation therapy have been reported. The potential for radiation related complication such as cataract, radiation optic neuropathy, and radiation retinopathy [57] exists, particularly in hemangiomas in the juxtapapillary and macular regions.

Diffuse Choroidal Hemangioma

About half the patients with Sturge-Weber syndrome have a diffuse choroidal hemangioma [58]. It is usually unilateral, and ipsilateral to the nevus flammeus [59]. Visual loss is due to refractive errors, foveal distortion, and exudative retinal detachment [42]. Although congenital in origin, choroidal hemangioma may not cause exudative retinal detachment until later in childhood or early adolescence [48].

Diagnosis

The choroidal hemangioma appears as diffuse choroidal thickening (tomato-catsup appearance of fundus) with or without associated exudative retinal detachment. Diagnostic techniques such as angiography, ultrasonography, and magnetic resonance imaging can be useful in confirming the clinical diagnosis.

Management of Primary Disease

The decision to treat should be individualized based upon the extent of symptoms, visual loss, and any potential for visual recovery. Asymptomatic cases, especially in the absence of an exudative retinal detachment, the hemangioma can be safely observed.

Schilling and associates reported their results on 15 eyes that were treated by lens sparing radiation (20 Gy, 10 fractions) with a mean follow-up of more than 5 years [50].

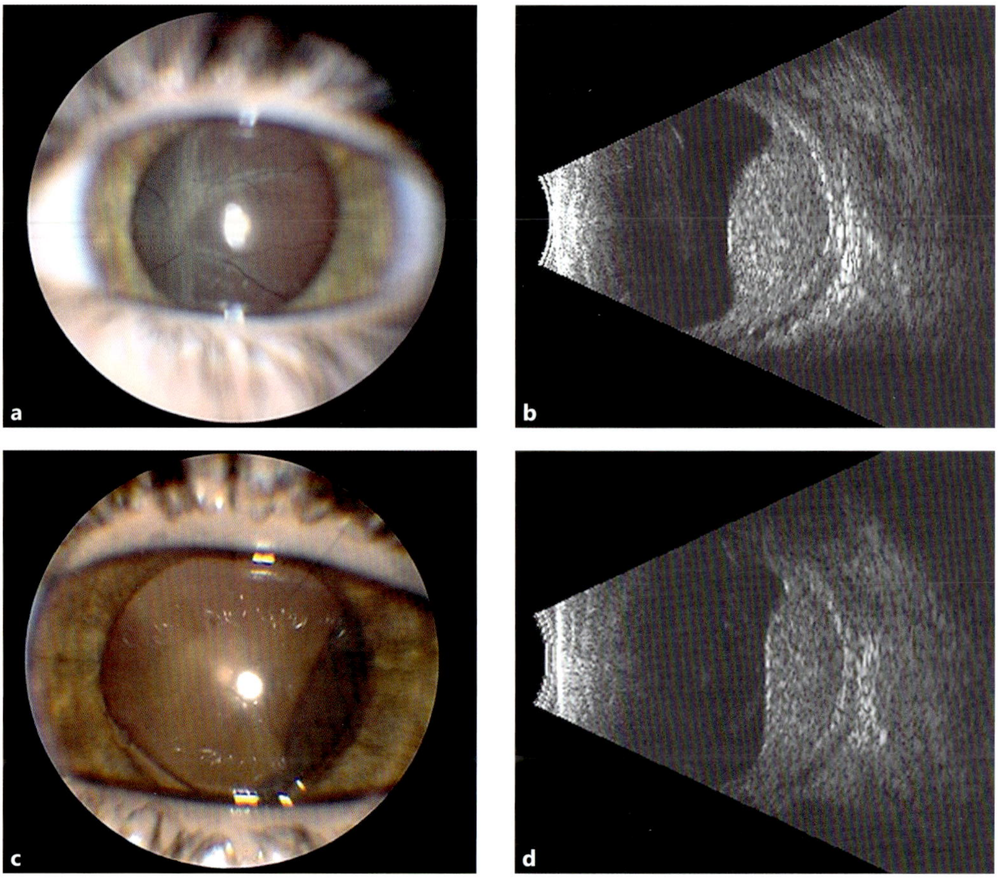

Fig. 5. A 14-year-old female complained of blurred vision out of her left eye. An ocular examination performed 2 years prior was unremarkable, except for anisometric amblyopia of her left eye. Past medical history included treatment for a port wine stain affecting the left V1 and V2 areas of her face. On examination, visual acuity was 20/20 in the right eye and light perception in the left eye. In the left eye the anterior chamber was shallow without rubeosis. Intraocular pressure was 22 mm Hg. Overall, the left fundus had an orange hue which was more evident superiorly than inferiorly. Fundus evaluation revealed total exudative retinal detachment with apposition of the retina to the posterior aspect of the lens (**a**). Ultrasound B-scan demonstrating a diffuse choroidal hemangioma with a localized prominence and a maximal height of 8.0 mm and an exudative retinal detachment (**b**). Six months posttreatment showing reattachment of the retina (**c**) and a reduction in maximal height to 6.0 mm (**d**).

Complete resolution of exudative retinal detachment in all cases, tumor regression in 5 cases, and improved vision in 7 eyes was observed (fig. 5). Zografos et al. [54] treated 6 diffuse hemangiomas in patients with Sturge-Weber syndrome with total proton dose ranging from 16.4 to 18.2 Gy applied in four daily fractions. Local tumor control and resolution of secondary retinal detachment was achieved in all cases. Kim et al. [60] reported excellent results in 7 patients with symptomatic choroidal hemangioma (4

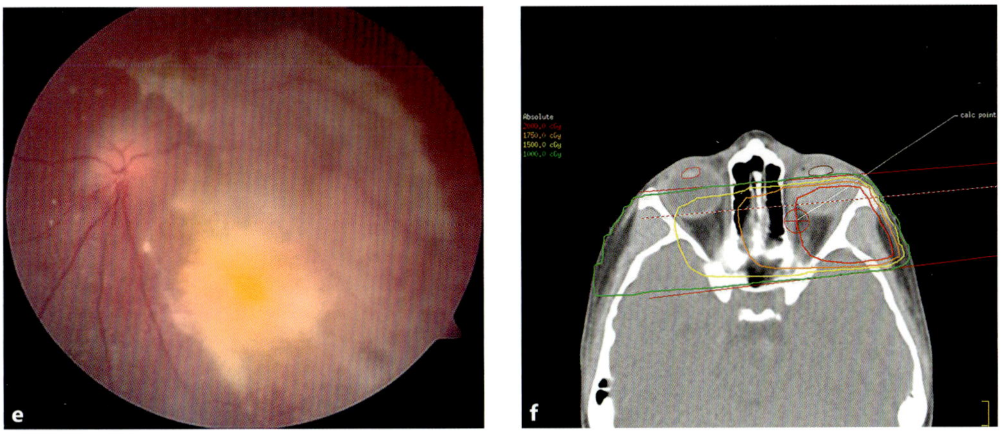

Fig. 5. One year posttreatment, demonstrating complete reattachment of retina with residual retinal folds (**e**). The patient was treated with a single left lateral radiation field using 6 MV photons prescribed to a depth of 4 cm (identified by the calc [calculation] point above). The field tilts posteriorly left-to-right to avoid treating the contralateral lens. The 2,000-, 1,750-, 1,500- and 1,000-cGy isodose lines are displayed (inside-outside). Note that the left and right eye lenses are not in the field of radiation (**f**). Reproduced with permission from Grant LW, Anderson C, Macklis RM, Singh AD: Low dose irradiation for diffuse choroidal hemangioma. Ophthal Genet 2008;29:186–188.

with diffuse form) were treated with the 10 Gy radiation delivered by the Leksell Gamma Knife. They observed resolution of exudative retinal detachment and improved visual acuity in all eyes.

Prognosis

Sturge-Weber syndrome with its neural involvement can cause intractable seizures, developmental delay and behavioral problems. Ocular manifestations including congenital glaucoma generally require multiple surgical procedures.

Uveal Lymphoma

Typically, this is a non-Hodgkin's lymphoma, most frequently of B cell origin. It can be classified as either primary uveal lymphoma or as a secondary intraocular manifestation of systemic lymphoma [61]. Histopathologically, uveal lymphoma may be one of several subtypes; extranodal marginal zone B cell lymphoma is the predominant form, comprising 60–80% of cases [62, 63]. Primary uveal lymphoma accounts for approximately 70–80 case reports and small case series in the literature [64, 65]. A strong correlation has been observed between uveal lymphoma and co-existing ocular adnexal lymphoma [66–68]. Uveal lymphoma may in fact be more accurately classified as a variant of ocular adnexal lymphoma [66].

Diagnosis

The dominant fundus finding was yellow-white choroidal infiltrates diffuse choroidal thickening, and evidence of extrascleral extension on B-scan ultrasonography.

Management of Primary Disease

Primary treatment selections included external beam radiotherapy (EBRT), rituximab, or rituximab combined with cyclophosphamide, hydroxydaunorubicin, oncovin and prednisone (RHCOP). The majority of patients are treated with EBRT, if they localized ophthalmic disease after detailed staging evaluation [see chapter 'Radiation Therapy: Orbital Tumors' by Marwaha et al., this vol.]. In a series of 18 patients, the median dose of radiation was 30 Gy (range 2,340–3,600 cGy) [69]. All patients (100%) with localized disease treated with EBRT achieved complete remission (median follow-up 28.7 months) (fig. 6).

Prognosis

Uveal lymphoma is most frequently low-grade and indolent in nature, therefore the clinical course is often less aggressive than in other forms of lymphoma with excellent overall survival [65].

Uveal Metastases

An estimated 8–10% of patients with metastatic malignancy have uveal involvement [70]. Therefore, metastasis is the most common uveal malignancy. Metastases usually involve the choroid (88% of cases) and rarely involve the iris (9% of cases) or ciliary body (2% of cases) [71]. Breast is the most common primary site in women and lung is the most common primary site in men [71–74]. In a large series of uveal metastases the distribution of primary sites included breast (47% of cases), lung (21% of cases), and GI tract (4% of cases) [71]. Interestingly, lung is the most likely primary site of uveal metastatic carcinoma in patients with no known primary at presentation [71, 75–78]. In contrast, uveal metastases from breast carcinoma usually occur late in the natural history and are associated with disseminated disease in patients with a known breast primary [73, 79]. Importantly, sarcomas rarely metastasize to the uvea [72].

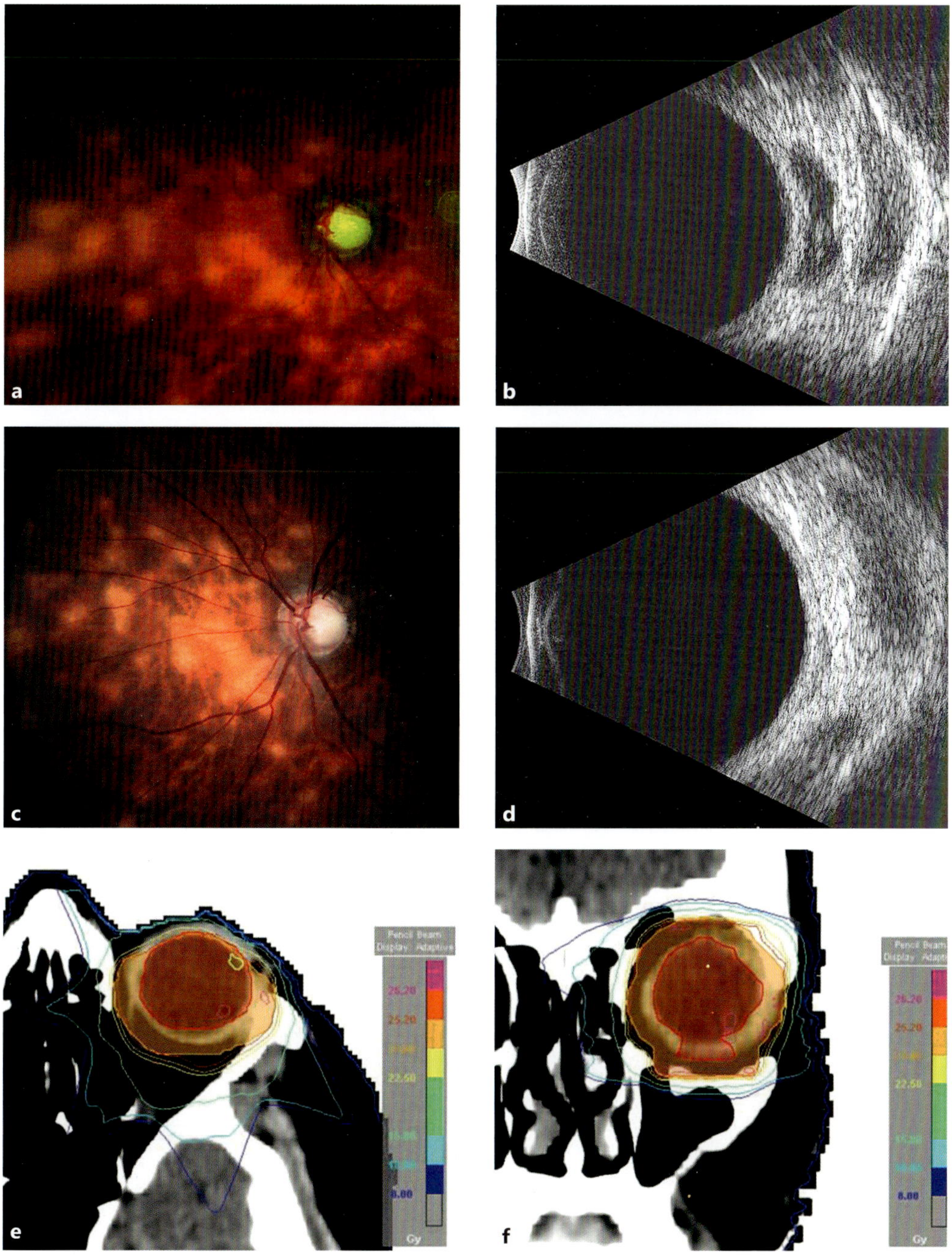

Fig. 6. A 70-year-old woman with blurred vision in the left eye of about 6 months' duration. There was mild proptosis. External examination revealed absence of salmon patch infiltration in both eyes. Right eye was normal. Fundus evaluation of the left eye showed focal infiltration of the posterior choroid, most prominent in the nasal quadrant (**a**). Ultrasonography showed diffuse choroidal infiltration. In addition, discrete extra scleral lesion was identified (**b**). Note total resolution of choroidal infiltration (**c**), and total resolution of orbital component (**d**) 3 months after radiation therapy – 6 MV photons via intensity modulated fields (axial (**e**) and coronal views (**f**), 2,520 cGY in 14 fractions of 180 cGy each).

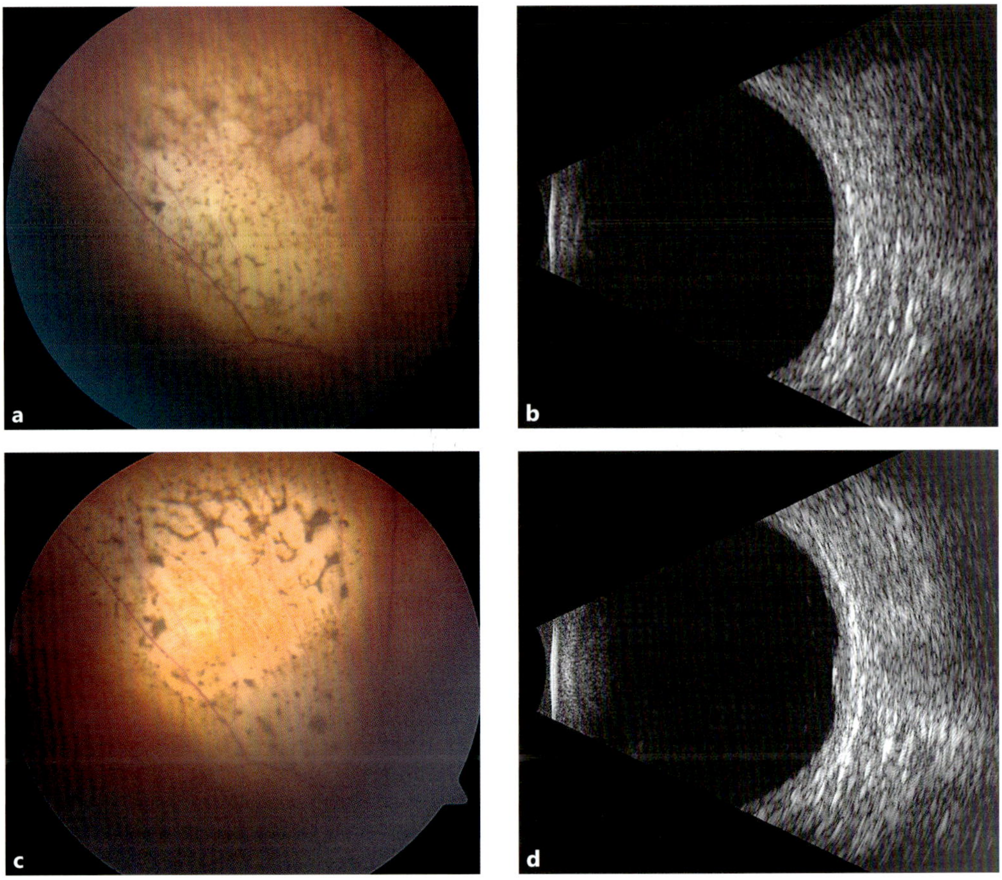

Fig. 7. A 79-year-old lady presented with visual disturbance in the right eye of a few months duration. The past history was significant for right breast lumpectomy followed by local radiotherapy 2 years prior. Although she was started on oral anostrazole, she developed blood clots requiring discontinuation of treatment. On examination, visual acuity was 20/50 in the right eye and 20/20 in the left eye (normal). Fundus evaluation of the right eye showed normal optic disc and macula. In the superior temporal quadrant, a circumscribed amelanotic choroidal lesion was identified (**a**). It was 8.5 × 7 mm in basal dimension with a thickness of about 1.5 mm (**b**). Smaller but distinct second lesion was also noted. Additional evaluation indicated presence of spinal metastasis. She was treated by external radiotherapy to the right eye (30 Gy in 15 fractions) and spinal lesion. 3 months later, there was definite evidence of tumor regression with only atrophic chorioretinal changes and overlying retinal pigment epithelial stippling (**c**) and flattening on ultrasonography (**d**).

Diagnosis

Multifocality and or bilaterality can help clinically differentiate metastases from primary tumors, especially melanoma. However, metastases are often solitary and unilateral [71, 73]. Diagnostic fine-needle aspiration biopsy (FNAB) is usually indicated in the work up of uveal metastases, especially when a primary malignancy is not known (approximately one third of patients) or in those rare cases with contentious clinical findings [72, 80–82].

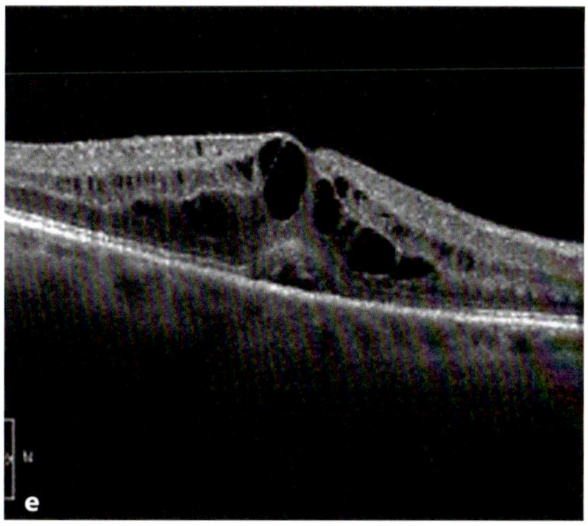

Fig. 7. About 1 year after the radiation therapy, visual acuity dropped to 20/200 due to radiation retinopathy (**e**, optical coherence tomography showing cystoid macular edema).

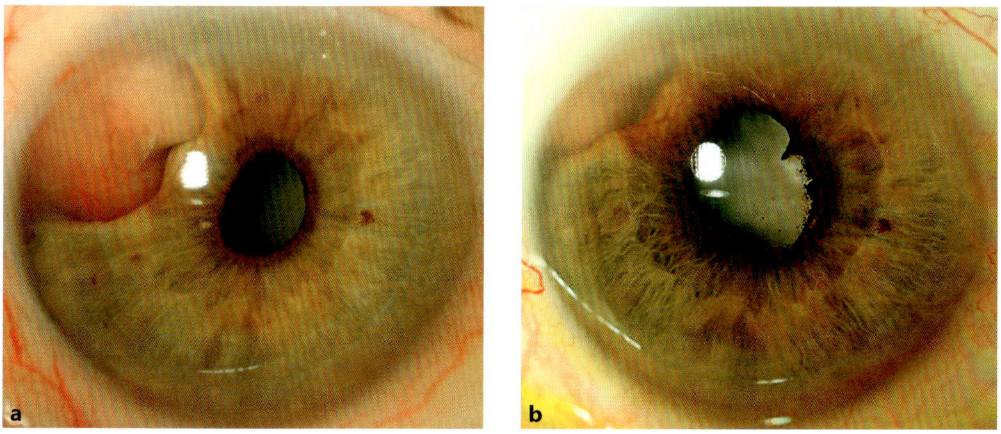

Fig. 8. A 68-year-old man initially presented with left hip pain which led to a diagnosis of left renal mass with widespread bone metastasis. Left radical nephrectomy showed evidence of clear cell type renal cell carcinoma (grade 4). There was evidence of penetration of the renal capsule and infiltration of perinephric fat and invasion of the renal vein. He was treated with interferon alpha, local radiation therapy, and zoledronic acid. He continued to progress slowly despite being treated with several investigational drugs developing ocular pain 4 years later. On examination visual acuity was 20/200 D with normal intraocular pressure. A kidney-shaped vascular mass was visible in the iridociliary region (**a**). Four weeks following treatment with iodine-125 plaque radiotherapy, marked regression of the lesion is evident (**b**). Reproduced with permission from Biscotti and Singh [82].

Management of Primary Disease

It is important to perform systemic evaluation to determine the extent of metastasis, particularly the involvement of the brain. If the metastatic disease is diffuse then the treatment options include chemotherapy, hormonal therapy (for hormone-dependent tumors), immune modulation, and angiogenic inhibitors depending upon the type of primary tumor and response to prior therapy [62]. Surgical treatment (enucleation) may be necessary for painful eyes with secondary glaucoma.

Radiation therapy is usually recommended for focal disease (confined to the uvea or orbit). The standard procedure of external beam radiation therapy makes use of asymmetric unilateral or bilateral fields generated by a linear accelerator, with a target volume dose of 35–40 Gy in 20 fractions (fig. 7) [see chapter 'Radiation Therapy: Orbital Tumors' by Marwaha et al., this vol.]. Although proton treatment is effective in treating choroidal metastases, there may not be justifiable benefit over external beam radiotherapy given the excessive cost of proton treatment [83]. Selected solitary metastatic tumors can be treated with a radioactive plaque, which has the advantage of a shorter interval and a more target-oriented delivery than external beam radiotherapy (fig. 8) [84, 85].

Prognosis

Using this approach, visual acuity can be improved or stabilized in 86% of patients [86]. Immediate complications of external beam therapy, such as erythema and conjunctivitis, are usually mild and transient [see chapter 'Radiation Therapy: Anterior Segment Complications' by Medina Mendez and Singh, this vol.]. As the overall survival rate is poor, late complications of radiation therapy, such as radiation retinopathy, are not experienced by most patients.

Conclusions

Management of primary uveal melanoma has been much improved during the past decades and most eyes with are now being retained with some visual function. Unfortunately, the prognosis of systemic uveal melanoma has not been similarly improved and almost half of patients with primary disease still die with metastatic spread. Most patients with primary disease receive some form of radiotherapy, although enucleation of the eye is still used for approximately a third of patients. Management of systemic disease is controversial with many experimental techniques being used. Experience gained from treating uveal melanoma has been expanded to treat benign uveal tumors such as choroidal hemangioma and other malignant tumors such as uveal lymphoma and uveal metastasis.

References

1 Singh AD, De Potter P, Fijal BA, et al: Lifetime prevalence of uveal melanoma in white patients with oculo(dermal) melanocytosis. Ophthalmology 1998;105:195–198.

2 Singh AD, Shields CL, Shields JA, De Potter P: Bilateral primary uveal melanoma. Bad luck or bad genes? Ophthalmology 1996;103:256–262.

3 Abdel-Rahman MH, Pilarski R, Cebulla CM, et al: Germline BAP1 mutation predisposes to uveal melanoma, lung adenocarcinoma, meningioma, and other cancers. J Med Genet 2011;48:856–859.

4 Carbone M, Ferris LK, Baumann F, et al: BAP1 cancer syndrome: malignant mesothelioma, uveal and cutaneous melanoma, and MBAITs. J Transl Med 2012;10:179.

5 Harbour JW: The genetics of uveal melanoma: an emerging framework for targeted therapy. Pigment Cell Melanoma Res 2012;25:171–181.

6 Bergman L, Seregard S, Nilsson B, et al: Incidence of uveal melanoma in Sweden from 1960 to 1998. Invest Ophthalmol Vis Sci 2002;43:2579–2583.

7 Singh AD, Turell ME, Topham AK: Uveal melanoma: trends in incidence, treatment, and survival. Ophthalmology 2011;118:1881–1885.

8 Lutz JM, Cree I, Sabroe S, et al: Occupational risks for uveal melanoma results from a case-control study in nine European countries. Cancer Causes Control 2005;16:437–447.

9 Cohen Y, Goldenberg-Cohen N, Parrella P, et al: Lack of BRAF mutation in primary uveal melanoma. Invest Ophthalmol Vis Sci 2003;44:2876–2878.

10 Cruz F 3rd, Rubin BP, Wilson D, et al: Absence of BRAF and NRAS mutations in uveal melanoma. Cancer Res 2003;63:5761–5766.

11 Kilic E, Bruggenwirth HT, Verbiest MM, et al: The RAS-BRAF kinase pathway is not involved in uveal melanoma. Melanoma Res 2004;14:203–205.

12 Singh AD, Rennie IG, Seregard S, et al: Sunlight exposure and pathogenesis of uveal melanoma. Surv Ophthalmol 2004;49:419–428.

13 Histopathologic characteristics of uveal melanomas in eyes enucleated from the Collaborative Ocular Melanoma Study. COMS report No. 6. Am J Ophthalmol 1998;125:745–766.

14 Midena E, Parrozzani R: Biopsies in uveal melanoma. Dev Ophthalmol 2012;49:81–95.

15 Damato EM, Damato BE: Detection and time to treatment of uveal melanoma in the United Kingdom: an evaluation of 2,384 patients. Ophthalmology 2012;119:1582–1589.

16 Shields CL, Furuta M, Berman EL, et al: Choroidal nevus transformation into melanoma: analysis of 2,514 consecutive cases. Arch Ophthalmol 2009;127:981–987.

17 Collaborative Ocular Melanoma Study G. The COMS randomized trial of iodine 125 brachytherapy for choroidal melanoma. V. Twelve-year mortality rates and prognostic factors: COMS report No. 28. Arch Ophthalmol 2006;124:1684–1693.

18 Collaborative Ocular Melanoma Study G. Trends in size and treatment of recently diagnosed choroidal melanoma, 1987–1997. Findings from patients examined at collaborative ocular melanoma study (COMS) centers: COMS report No. 20. Arch Ophthalmol 2003;121:1156–1162.

19 Wilkinson DA, Kolar M, Fleming PA, Singh AD: Dosimetric comparison of 106Ru and 125I plaques for treatment of shallow (< or = 5 mm) choroidal melanoma lesions. Br J Radiol 2008;81:784–789.

20 Bergman L, Nilsson B, Lundell G, et al: Ruthenium brachytherapy for uveal melanoma, 1979–2003: survival and functional outcomes in the Swedish population. Ophthalmology 2005;112:834–840.

21 Damato B, Patel I, Campbell IR, et al: Local tumor control after 106Ru brachytherapy of choroidal melanoma. Int J Radiat Oncol Biol Phys 2005;63:385–391.

22 Gragoudas ES, Marie Lane A: Uveal melanoma: proton beam irradiation. Ophthalmol Clin North Am 2005;18:111–118, ix.

23 Damato BE: Local resection of uveal melanoma. Dev Ophthalmol 2012;49:66–80.

24 Zehetmayer M: Stereotactic photon beam irradiation of uveal melanoma. Dev Ophthalmol 2012;49:58–65.

25 Singh AD, Kivela T, Seregard S, et al: Primary transpupillary thermotherapy of 'small' choroidal melanoma: is it safe? Br J Ophthalmol 2008;92:727–728.

26 Damato B: Progress in the management of patients with uveal melanoma. The 2012 Ashton Lecture. Eye (Lond) 2012;26:1157–1172.

27 Diener-West M, Reynolds SM, Agugliaro DJ, et al: Screening for metastasis from choroidal melanoma: the Collaborative Ocular Melanoma Study Group Report 23. J Clin Oncol 2004;22:2438–2444.

28 Mouriaux F, Diorio C, Bergeron D, et al: Liver function testing is not helpful for early diagnosis of metastatic uveal melanoma. Ophthalmology 2012;119:1590–1595.

29 Brandberg Y, Kock E, Oskar K, et al: Psychological reactions and quality of life in patients with posterior uveal melanoma treated with ruthenium plaque therapy or enucleation: a one year follow-up study. Eye (Lond) 2000;14:839–846.

30 Melia M, Moy CS, Reynolds SM, et al: Quality of life after iodine 125 brachytherapy vs enucleation for choroidal melanoma: 5-year results from the Collaborative Ocular Melanoma Study: COMS QOLS Report No. 3. Arch Ophthalmol 2006;124:226–238.

31 Singh AD, Topham A: Survival rates with uveal melanoma in the United States: 1973–1997. Ophthalmology 2003;110:962–965.
32 Singh AD, Borden EC: Metastatic uveal melanoma. Ophthalmol Clin North Am 2005;18:143–150, ix.
33 Bergman L, Seregard S, Nilsson B, et al: Uveal melanoma survival in Sweden from 1960 to 1998. Invest Ophthalmol Vis Sci 2003;44:3282–3287.
34 Kujala E, Makitie T, Kivela T: Very long-term prognosis of patients with malignant uveal melanoma. Invest Ophthalmol Vis Sci 2003;44:4651–4659.
35 Singh AD: Uveal melanoma: implications of tumor doubling time. Ophthalmology 2001;108:829–831.
36 Seregard S, Kock E: Prognostic indicators following enucleation for posterior uveal melanoma. A multivariate analysis of long-term survival with minimized loss to follow-up. Acta Ophthalmol Scand 1995;73:340–344.
37 Seregard S, Oskarsson M, Spangberg B: PC-10 as a predictor of prognosis after antigen retrieval in posterior uveal melanoma. Invest Ophthalmol Vis Sci 1996;37:1451–1458.
38 Seregard S, Spangberg B, Juul C, Oskarsson M: Prognostic accuracy of the mean of the largest nucleoli, vascular patterns, and PC-10 in posterior uveal melanoma. Ophthalmology 1998;105:485–491.
39 Prescher G, Bornfeld N, Becher R: Nonrandom chromosomal abnormalities in primary uveal melanoma. J Natl Cancer Inst 1990;82:1765–1769.
40 Aalto Y, Eriksson L, Seregard S, et al: Concomitant loss of chromosome 3 and whole arm losses and gains of chromosome 1, 6, or 8 in metastasizing primary uveal melanoma. Invest Ophthalmol Vis Sci 2001;42:313–317.
41 Onken MD, Worley LA, Ehlers JP, Harbour JW: Gene expression profiling in uveal melanoma reveals two molecular classes and predicts metastatic death. Cancer Res 2004;64:7205–7209.
42 Anand R, Augsburger JJ, Shields JA: Circumscribed choroidal hemangiomas. Arch Ophthalmol 1989; 107:1338–1342.
43 Shields CL, Honavar SG, Shields JA, et al: Circumscribed choroidal hemangioma: clinical manifestations and factors predictive of visual outcome in 200 consecutive cases. Ophthalmology 2001;108:2237–2248.
44 Witschel H, Font RL: Hemangioma of the choroid. A clinicopathologic study of 71 cases and a review of the literature. Surv Ophthalmol 1976;20:415–431.
45 Stroszczynski C, Hosten N, Bornfeld N, et al: Choroidal hemangioma: MR findings and differentiation from uveal melanoma. AJNR 1998;19:1441–1447.
46 Gunduz K: Transpupillary thermotherapy in the management of circumscribed choroidal hemangioma. Surv Ophthalmol 2004;49:316–327.
47 Singh AD, Kaiser PK, Sears JE, et al: Photodynamic therapy of circumscribed choroidal haemangioma. Br J Ophthalmol 2004;88:1414–1418.
48 Tsipursky MS, Golchet PR, Jampol LM: Photodynamic therapy of choroidal hemangioma in Sturge-Weber syndrome, with a review of treatments for diffuse and circumscribed choroidal hemangiomas. Surv Ophthalmol 2011;56:68–85.
49 Singh AD: Ocular phototherapy. Eye 2012;27:190–198.
50 Schilling H, Sauerwein W, Lommatzsch A: Long term results after low dose ocular irradiation for choproidal hemangioma. Br J Ophthalmol 1997;81:267–273.
51 Kivela T, Tenhunen M, Joensuu T, et al: Stereotactic radiotherapy of symptomatic circumscribed choroidal hemangiomas. Ophthalmology 2003;110:1977–1982.
52 Singh AD, Kaiser PK, Sears JE: Choroidal hemangioma. Ophthalmol Clin North Am 2005;18:151–161, ix.
53 Aizman A, Finger PT, Shabto U, et al: Palladium 103 (^{103}Pd) plaque radiation therapy for circumscribed choroidal hemangioma with retinal detachment. Arch Ophthalmol 2004;122:1652–1656.
54 Zografos L, Egger E, Bercher L, et al: Proton beam irradiation of choroidal hemangiomas. Am J Ophthalmol 1998;126:261–268.
55 Frau E, Rumen F, Noel G, et al: Low-dose proton beam therapy for circumscribed choroidal hemangiomas. Arch Ophthalmol 2004;122:1471–1475.
56 Nam TK, Lee JI, Kang SW: Gamma knife radiosurgery for circumscribed choroidal hemangioma. Acta Neurochir (Wien) 2005;147:651–654.
57 Zografos L, Bercher L, Chamot L, et al: Cobalt-60 treatment of choroidal hemangiomas. Am J Ophthalmol 1996;121:190–199.
58 Sullivan TJ, Clarke MP, Morin JD: The ocular manifestations of the Sturge-Weber syndrome. J Pediatr Ophthalmol Strabismus 1992;29:349–356.
59 Amirikia A, Scott IU, Murray TG: Bilateral diffuse choroidal hemangiomas with unilateral facial nevus flammeus in Sturge-Weber syndrome. Am J Ophthalmol 2000;130:362–364.
60 Kim YT, Kang SW, Lee JI: Gamma knife radiosurgery for choroidal hemangioma. Int J Radiat Oncol Biol Phys 2011;81:1399–1404.
61 Thieblemont C, Coiffier B: Management of marginal zone lymphomas. Curr Treatm Options Oncol 2006; 7:213–222.
62 Bornfeld N: Uveal metastatic tumors; in Singh AD, Damato BE, Pe'er J, et al (eds): Clinical Ophthalmic Oncology. Philadelphia, Saunders-Elsevier, 2007.
63 Freeman C, Berg JW, Cutler SJ: Occurrence and prognosis of extranodal lymphomas. Cancer 1972; 29:252–260.
64 Coupland SE: Uveal Lymphoproliferative Tumors; in Singh AD, Damato BE, Pe'er J, et al (eds): Clinical Ophthalmic Oncology. Philadelphia, Saunders-Elsevier, 2007.

65 Coupland SE, Joussen A, Anastassiou G, Stein H: Diagnosis of a primary uveal extranodal marginal zone B-cell lymphoma by chorioretinal biopsy: case report. Graefe's Arch Clin Exp Ophthalmol 2005;243:482–486.
66 Fuller ML, Sweetenham J, Schoenfield L, Singh AD: Uveal lymphoma: a variant of ocular adnexal lymphoma. Leukemia Lymphoma 2008;49:2393–2397.
67 Grossniklaus HE, Martin DF, Avery R, et al: Uveal lymphoid infiltration. Report of four cases and clinicopathologic review. Ophthalmology 1998;105:1265–1273.
68 Sarraf D, Jain A, Dubovy S, et al: Mucosa-associated lymphoid tissue lymphoma with intraocular involvement. Retina 2005;25:94–98.
69 Aronow ME, Portell CA, Sweetenham JW, Singh AD: Uveal lymphoma: clinical features, diagnostic studies, treatment selection, and outcomes. Ophthalmology, in press.
70 Wickremasinghe S, Dansingani KK, Tranos P, et al: Ocular presentations of breast cancer. Acta Ophthalmol Scand 2007;85:133–142.
71 Shields CL, Shields JA, Gross NE, et al: Survey of 520 eyes with uveal metastases. Ophthalmology 1997;104:1265–1276.
72 Shields JA, Shields CL, Kiratli H, de Potter P: Metastatic tumors to the iris in 40 patients. Am J Ophthalmol 1995;119:422–430.
73 Soysal HG: Metastatic tumors of the uvea in 38 eyes. Can J Ophthalmol 2007;42:832–835.
74 Lam A, Shields CL, Shields JA: Uveal metastases from breast carcinoma in three male patients. Ophthalmic Surg Lasers Imaging 2006;37:320–323.
75 Kreusel KM, Bechrakis NE, Wiegel T, et al: Incidence and clinical characteristics of symptomatic choroidal metastasis from lung cancer. Acta Ophthalmol 2008;86:515–519.
76 Bandyopadhyay S, Adrean SD, Puklin JE, Feng J: Choroidal metastasis from an occult primary diagnosed by fine-needle aspiration: a case report. Diagn Cytopathol 2009;37:38–41.
77 Trichopoulos N, Augsburger JJ: Neuroendocrine tumours metastatic to the uvea: diagnosis by fine needle aspiration biopsy. Graefes Arch Clin Exp Ophthalmol 2006;244:524–528.
78 John VJ, Jacobson MS, Grossniklaus HE: Bilateral choroidal metastasis as the presenting sign of small cell lung carcinoma. J Thorac Oncol 2010;5:1289.
79 Kreusel KM, Bechrakis NE, Krause L, et al: Incidence and clinical characteristics of symptomatic choroidal metastasis from breast cancer. Acta Ophthalmol Scand 2007;85:298–302.
80 Augsburger JJ: Fine needle aspiration biopsy of suspected metastatic cancers to the posterior uvea. Trans Am Ophthalmol Soc 1988;86:499–560.
81 Kanthan GL, Jayamohan J, Yip D, Conway RM: Management of metastatic carcinoma of the uveal tract: an evidence-based analysis. Clin Exp Ophthalmol 2007;35:553–565.
82 Biscotti CV, Singh AD: Uveal metastases. Monogr Clin Cytol 2012;21:17–30.
83 Tsina EK, Lane AM, Zacks DN, et al: Treatment of metastatic tumors of the choroid with proton beam irradiation. Ophthalmology 2005;112:337–343.
84 Lim JI, Petrovich Z: Radioactive plaque therapy for metastatic choroidal carcinoma. Ophthalmology 2000;107:1927–1931.
85 Shields CL, Shields JA, De Potter P, et al: Plaque radiotherapy for the management of uveal metastasis. Arch Ophthalmol 1997;115:203–209.
86 Wiegel T, Bottke D, Kreusel KM, et al: External beam radiotherapy of choroidal metastases – final results of a prospective study of the German Cancer Society (ARO 95–08). Radiother Oncol 2002;64:13–18.

Stefan Seregard, MD
St Eriks Eye Hospital, Karolinska Institutet
Polhemsgatan 50
SE–11 282 Stockholm (Sweden)
E-Mail stefan.seregard@sankterik.se

Singh AD, Pelayes DE, Seregard S, Macklis R (eds): Ophthalmic Radiation Therapy. Techniques and Applications.
Dev Ophthalmol. Basel, Karger, 2013, vol 52, pp 58–74 (DOI: 10.1159/000351058)

Radiation Therapy: Retinal Tumors

Roshan V. Sethi[a] · Shannon M. MacDonald[a] · David Y. Kim[b] · Shizuo Mukai[b]

[a]Department of Radiation Oncology, Massachusetts General Hospital and [b]Department of Ophthalmology, Massachusetts Eye and Ear Infirmary, Harvard Medical School, Boston, Mass., USA

Abstract

The major retinal tumor that requires radiotherapy (RT) is retinoblastoma (RB); to a lesser degree, RT is used for some cases of retinal capillary hemangioma and lymphoma of the retina. Although there are concerns about the risk of RT-induced second malignancy in patients who carry a germline mutation in the *RB1* gene, RT remains a very important part of our approach to intra-ocular and extra-ocular RB. Technical innovations in RT allow more precise targeting of retinal tumors and decreased exposure of adjacent normal tissue, an advance that is particularly significant for patients with hereditary RB who are at risk of additional malignancies.

Retinoblastoma

Retinoblastoma (RB) is a rare primary intraocular tumor with an incidence of approximately one in 20,000 births. Survival from RB is above 90% with modern treatment methods. Approximately one-third of cases carry a germline mutation in the *RB1* gene, and this is significant for radiotherapy (RT) since carriers are at increased risk for second malignancies and that risk is increased with radiation exposure. Despite the relatively low mortality rate from RB, approximately 25% of hereditary RB survivors die of a second cancer, particularly osteosarcomas and soft tissue sarcomas, by age 50 years [1]. Because of this risk, RT has been largely replaced by upfront chemotherapy in patients with early stage disease. RT continues to be important in cases of advanced and chemo-refractory disease [2].

Table 1. International classification for intraocular retinoblastoma

Group A: very low risk Small tumors away from foveola and disc ≤3 mm in size, ≥3 mm from the foveola, ≥1.5 mm from the optic nerve No vitreous or subretinal seeding
Group B: low risk Any size or location tumor not in group A No vitreous/subretinal seeding Cuff of subretinal fluid ≤5 mm
Group C: moderate risk Any size or location tumor not in group A–B Focal vitreous or subretinal seeding No more than one quadrant of subretinal fluid
Group D: high risk Massive nondiscrete endophytic or exophytic tumors and/or diffuse vitreous or subretinal seeding
Group E: very high risk Irreversible neovascular glaucoma, massive intraocular hemorrhage, aseptic orbital cellulitis, tumor anterior to anterior vitreous face, tumor touching lens Diffuse infiltrating retinoblastoma Phthsis or prephthisis

The grouping and staging system for RB has evolved significantly in the past two decades. The Reese-Ellsworth (RE) classification scheme predicted local control after external beam radiation therapy (EBRT) [3]. In 2005, Linn Murphree [4] proposed the International Classification for Intraocular Retinoblastoma (ICIR) (table 1) that organizes tumors by characteristics that predict the need for enucleation or EBRT after upfront chemoreduction. It is now widely used instead of the RE classification, but neither scheme addressed extraocular disease. In 2006, Chantada et al. [5] proposed a staging system for extraocular RB that is used in the Children's Oncology Group (COG) extraocular RB protocol, ARET 0321.

Radiotherapy of Retinoblastoma

Radiotherapy is most commonly used in cases of intraocular RB that are refractory to chemotherapy (either systemic or intra-arterial) combined with laser and/or cryotherapy. It is sometimes used as primary therapy when small tumors involve the fovea or there is a high likelihood of needing RT following chemotherapy. Some centers consider failure of a chemotherapy-based treatment as total failure, avoid RT and

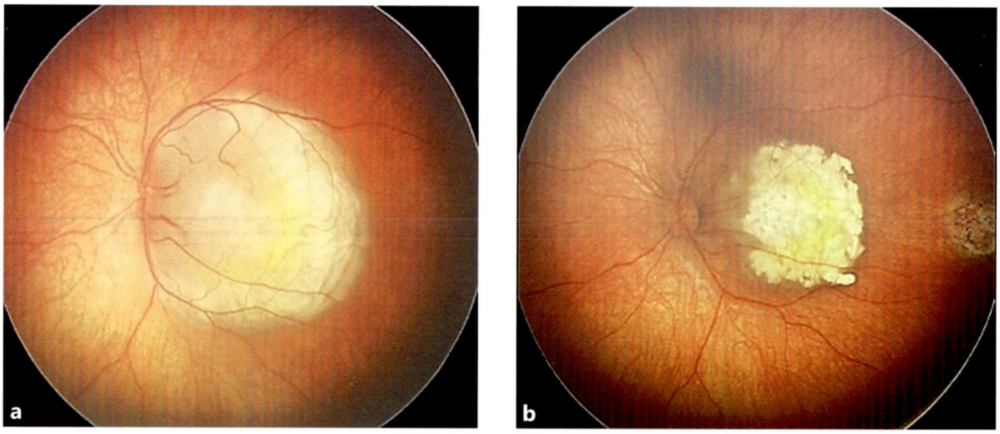

Fig. 1. 6-month-old child with a unilateral single juxtapilllary retinoblastoma, without evidence of optic nerve extension or seeding (**a**). 4 weeks after treatment with a notched iodine-125 plaque (total apical dose of 45 Gy delivered over 48 h) note satisfactory regression of the tumor (**b**). Even after 4 years, the tumor continues to demonstrate stable regression. Courtesy of Arun D. Singh, MD, Cleveland, Ohio, USA.

proceed to enucleation. We do not advocate this approach. External-beam RT (including stereotactic RT, intensity-modulated RT (IMRT), proton RT) is usually indicated in extraocular disease.

Radiotherapy of Intraocular Retinoblastoma

Brachytherapy

Brachytherapy techniques are described in detail in the chapter 'Brachytherapy' by Marwaha et al. [this vol.]. Tumors between 6 and 18 mm in height are considered suitable for brachytherapy [6–10]. Proximity to the optic nerve within 2 mm is contraindicated, but 'notching' of the radioactive plaque may allow successful treatment of lesions located close to the optic nerve (fig. 1) [8, 9]. Iodine-125 (^{125}I) and ruthenium-106 (^{106}Ru) are the commonly used sources. Plaques are sized with a margin of 1–2 mm around the tumor. A dose rate between 0.4 and 0.8 Gy/h is delivered with total doses to the tumor apex of 30–45 Gy over the course of 2–5 days [6–10]. The efficacy of ^{125}I plaque as primary treatment for RB and as focal therapy after chemoreduction is well established [6–9]. Shields et al. [8] reviewed the outcomes of 84 tumors in 71 eyes that received upfront chemoreduction followed by ^{125}I plaque brachytherapy. The tumor recurrence rate at 5 years was 5%. The complication rate was high with 27% of patients developing nonproliferative retinopathy [8]. Other complications were proliferative retinopathy, maculopathy and cataract. The complications increased with prior chemotherapy and higher rate and dose delivered to the tumor [8, 9].

External Beam Radiation Therapy

Radiation therapy was first used to treat RB in 1903 [11]. Until less than 15 years ago, RT was the primary, often definitive, treatment for RB [12–15]. Cassady et al. [13] reported that of 223 eyes treated by primary EBRT, 154 (69%) were spared enucleation and nearly all eyes (96%) available for testing had fair-to-good visual function. With recent techniques, ocular salvage rates of RE I–III eyes were between 81 and 100% and in RE IV–V eyes between 60 and 79% (table 2) [6, 16–26].

Several considerations enter into the decision to use EBRT which is most often used to salvage eyes with progressive or persistent disease after chemotherapy and focal therapy. The potential for vision is the most important as radiation may be able to best preserve vision [27]. Age at treatment less than 12 months increases the risk of second malignancy and age younger than 6 months substantially increases the risk of orbital hypoplasia [28]. Larger and thicker tumors are less likely to respond to chemotherapy and focal therapy [29]. In addition, focal therapy is more likely to cause permanent visual loss when used on tumors close to the macula and optic nerve. Radiotherapy, however, can treat tumors in these sensitive locations with the least impact on vision [15, 29, 30].

The final consideration is advanced intraocular disease. Current chemotherapy regimens have limited efficacy in advanced intraocular disease, because most agents do not enter the vitreous or subretinal spaces effectively. Radiotherapy can accomplish ocular salvage in a majority of RE IV–V eyes (table 2). Abramson et al. [20] reviewed the outcomes of 63 RE Vb eyes and found that primary RT prevented enucleation in 60% (38/63) of eyes. The majority of preserved eyes had at least counting fingers vision. Most studies, however, continue to recommend upfront chemoreduction for advanced intraocular disease in the hope of avoiding RT in approximately 50% of RE V eyes [29]. It remains unclear whether avoidance of RT in an attempt to prevent its complications outweighs the complications of chemotherapy including toxicity, unknown effect on the rate of secondary malignancy and delay to RT [2, 31].

Radiotherapy for Extraocular Retinoblastoma

Stage II and III Disease

Eyes with tumor present on histopathology at the surgical margin of the optic nerve or outside of the sclera (stage II) should be treated with systemic chemotherapy followed by orbital RT (including the optic nerve up to the chiasm in cases with a positive optic nerve margin) to a dose of approximately 45 Gy [2, 17, 32, 33]. Frank extraocular disease confined to the orbit with or without involvement of the preauricular and cervical nodes is defined as locoregional disease [32]. Patients with locoregional disease should undergo neoadjuvant chemotherapy followed by enucleation and orbital irradiation with a dose between 40 and 50 Gy [2, 17, 32, 33]. For stage II and III

Table 2. Efficacy of primary radiation therapy for intraocular disease in recent series (1980– present)

Study	Number of eyes	Mean/median follow-up (range), months	Study years	Bilateral technique*	Mean/median dose range; dose per fraction, Gy	Eyes with local control, %[†]	Ocular salvage, % (nonactuarial)[‡]	Visual outcome
Hernandez et al. [22]	34	35.2 (12–93)	1980–1991	anterior and lateral wedged pair without lens block, 4–6 MV LA photon	44.3 (34.5–49.5); 1.5–2.0			14/25 with cataracts
RE I–II						11/14 (78.5)	–	
RE III–V						4/20 (20)	–	
All						15/34 (44)	25/34 (74)	
Pradhan et al. [17]	64	48.5	1976–1993	anterior and lateral wedged pair without lens block, 6–8 MV LA photon	42.27 (30–45.25); 9–26 fractions			useful or full vision
RE Ia						–	4/4 (100)	4/4 (100)
RE Ib						–	3/3 (100)	3/3 (100)
RE IIa						–	2/2 (100)	2/2 (100)
RE IIb						–	4/4 (100)	4/4 (100)
RE IIIa						–	1/2 (50)	1/2 (50)
RE IIIb						–	3/6 (50)	3/6 (50)
RE IVa						–	2/2 (100)	2/2 (100)
RE IVb						–	8/13 (62)	8/13 (61.5)
RE Va						–	10/13 (77)	6/13 (46.1)
RE Vb						–	5/15 (33)	1/15 (6.7)
All						22/64 (34.4)	42/64 (66)	34/64 (53.1) 17/64 (27) with cataracts
Blach et al. [21]	67	101 (13–159)	1979–1984	anterior lens-sparing, photon and electron beam	38–50; 2.5			
RE I–III						(37)[§]	(81)	22% with cataracts
RE IV–V						(34)	(60)	
All						(38)	(71)	
Blach et al. [21]	113	52 (4–108)	1984–1991	modified lateral beam, photon	42–46; 2			22% with cataracts
RE I-III						(84)	(94)	
RE IV–V						(50)	(61)	
All						(65)	(78)	
Schipper et al. [19]	54	72 (24–144)	1971–1982	lateral D-shaped beam, photon 6-8 MV LA	45; 3			
RE I						8/14 (57)	14/14 (100)	43/45 (95) were HM or greater
RE II						6/9 (67)	9/9 (100)	18/54 with cataracts
RE III						2/12 (17)	10/12 (83)	
RE IV**						3/14 (21)	11/14 (79)	
RE Va						3/5 (60)	0/5 (0)	
All						22/54 (41)	45/54 (81)	
Amendola et al. [7]	13	35 (5–93)	1975–1988	anterior and lateral oblique wedged pair, 6 meV LA	40–45; 1.5–2.0			8/11 with useful vision 5/11 with cataracts
RE IIa						–	2/2 (100)	
RE IIb						–	2/2 (100)	
RE IIIa						–	2/2 (100)	
RE IVa						–	1/2 (50)	
RE Vb						–	2/3 (67)	
All						–	11/13	

Table 2. Continued

Study	Number of eyes	Mean/median follow-up (range), months	Study years	Bilateral technique*	Mean/median dose range; dose per fraction, Gy	Eyes with local control, %†	Ocular salvage,% (nonactuarial)‡	Visual outcome
Merchant et al. [24]	49	88.6 (34.3–372.5)	1978–1998	anterior field en face, 12 MeV, electrons	36 (32–38)			–
RE I–II						–	23/24 (96)	
RE III–V						–	13/20 (65)††	
All						30/49 (61)	43/49 (88)	
Abramson et al. [15]	63		1979–2002	not specified	42–46; 1.8–2			24/28 (86) with HM or greater
RE Vb						31/63 (49)	38/63 (60)	24/63 (38.1) with cataracts
Hungerford et al. [23]	175	108 (24–204)	1970–1985	whole eye technique, lateral beam, LA, photon	35–44; 2–3.9			140/140 cataracts
RE I						14/16 (88)	16/16 (100)	
RE II						31/55 (56)	46/55 (84)	
RE III						40/68 (59)	56/68 (82)	
RE IV						1/7 (14)	3/7 (43)	
RE V						13/29 (45)	19/29 (66)	
All						99/175 (57)	140/175 (80)	
Toma et al. [26]	67	35 (12–82)	1986–1992	lateral 'Schipper' technique, 6 MV LA photon	40; 2			1/67 with cataracts
RE I						14/18 (78)	18/18 (100)	
RE II						22/33 (67)	29/33 (88)	
RE III						7/11 (64)	10/11 (91)	
RE IV						5/5 (100)	5/5 (100)	
All						48/67 (72)	62/67 (93)	
Scott et al. [25]	32	36 (7–72)	1989–1996	modified lateral beam, LA, photon	48 (44–54)			(37) with cataracts
RE I–III						(58)‡‡	–	
RE IV–V						(51)	(83)	
All						–	–	
Scott et al. [25]	26	39 (5–74)	1989–1996	relative lens-sparing, LA, photon	45 (36–49)			(16.9) with cataracts
RE I–III						(90)	–	
RE IV–V						(81)	(88)	
All						–	–	

RE = Reese-Ellsworth Classification (see table 1); LA = linear accelerator; MV = megavoltage; HM = hand motion.
* Refers to the technique and energy used in the majority of patients.
† Number of patients treated with EBRT alone; excludes focal techniques, chemotherapy and plaque radiotherapy.
‡ Patients who underwent enucleation and/or died of metastatic disease.
§ Local control and eye survival rates in both series by Blach et al. [21] were calculated using actuarial technique at 8 years.
** Two eyes were classified as RE IV despite vitreous seeding; both eyes were cured.
†† Five eyes had an unknown RE classification.
‡‡ Local control, eye survival and cataract formation rates in both series by Scott et al. [25] were calculated using the Kaplan-Meier method at 3 years.

disease, the COG protocol ARET 0321 administers induction chemotherapy followed by EBRT up to 45 Gy to the orbit, enlarged nodes, and chiasm.

Stage IVa and IVb Disease

Metastatic disease in the CNS (stage IVa) is thought to occur via spread through the optic nerve. The prognosis is dismal [34]. Patients are treated with intravenous and intrathecal chemotherapy. Craniospinal irradiation (CSI) may be administered for children over the age of three years despite the substantial risk of neurocognitive deficits and second malignancy. Doses to the craniospinal axis range between 18 and 36 Gy, followed by a boost of 10–15 Gy to measurable sites of disease [32, 34].

Non-CNS metastatic disease (stage IVb) also has a very poor prognosis. The most frequent sites of metastatic disease are bone and liver [35]. Systemic chemotherapy is followed by RT to metastatic sites. Dunkel et al. [36] recommended doses of 19.5 Gy to liver metastases and 30 Gy to bone metastases. There has been recent success with high-dose induction chemotherapy followed by autologous hematopoietic stem cell transplant [37].

For stage IVa and IVb disease, COG ARET 0321 administers neoadjuvant induction and consolidation therapy followed by autologous hematopoietic stem cell transplant. Radiotherapy is administered if metastatic disease shows less than a complete response. For stage IVa disease, metastatic lesions are treated to 36 Gy (except for pulmonary and diffuse abdominal involvement). For stage IVb disease, a CSI dose of 23.4 Gy (for patients below the age of 60 months) or 36 Gy (for patients above the age of 60 months) are recommended with involved field boosts between 36 and 50.4 Gy depending on the location.

Trilateral Disease

Trilateral disease refers to the development of a primitive neuroectodermal tumor in the pineal region (usually pinealoblastoma) with bilateral RB. It is considered a separate malignancy, not a metastatic lesion. Before the advent of upfront chemoreduction protocols, trilateral disease occurred in 6% of patients with bilateral RB and 10% if family history was also positive [38]. In the past, this was treated with CSI and chemotherapy [38]. COG ARET 0321 treats trilateral disease with the same protocol as metastatic disease involving the CNS (see above). Despite poor prognosis, several cases have been successfully treated using high-dose chemotherapy followed by autologous hematopoietic stem cell transplant and focal RT to the primitive neuroectodermal tumor [39].

External Beam Radiation Therapy Techniques for Retinoblastoma

Volume

In bilateral RB and in patients with a family history, a new tumor may develop anywhere in the retina [15]. Hernandez et al. [22] found that 23% of recurrences after RT occurred at a new site in previously uninvolved retina. For this reason, the entire retina was traditionally included in the target volume. In cases of vitreous seeding, the whole vitreous is included in the target volume [15]. Recently, with more precise teletherapy techniques such as proton RT and IMRT, we target the identifiable tumors and do not attempt 'prophylaxis' of uninvolved retina. We believe that laser and/or cryotherapy can effectively treat new tumors. This approach is not widely used, but the rationale is discussed in further detail in the following text.

Dose and Fractionation

Most institutions use a dose of 40 and 46 Gy to the clinical tumor volume with fractions between 1.8 and 2.0 Gy per day (table 2). Lower doses may be adequate, but are not widely used. Cassaday et al. [13] found no significant difference in local tumor control with 32–35 versus 40–45 Gy (41 vs. 53%). Similarly, Merchant et al. [24] showed that of 49 eyes treated at St. Jude's Children's Hospital with 32–38 Gy (median 36 Gy), the rates of ocular salvage (66% for RE III–V and 95% for RE I–II at 5 years) were similar to those that had been treated at a higher dose. Nevertheless, most institutions continue to treat to 40–46 Gy, partly because most patients currently referred for RT have advanced and treatment-refractory disease.

Hypofractionation increases the risk for RT complications, particularly retinopathy and cataract [17, 19, 40, 41]. Coucke et al. [40] found the risk of retinopathy to be associated significantly with dose per fraction, substantially increased above 2.5 Gy. Pradhan et al. [17] treated to 45 Gy with 3.75 Gy/fraction to limit exposure to anesthesia, and reported high rates of retinopathy, vitreous hemorrhage, glaucoma, and optic neuropathy in half of the 192 eyes treated. Most centers currently use fractions between 1.8 and 2.0 Gy.

Patient Set-Up

At our institution, patients are treated in the supine position under general anesthesia (i.v. propofol drip) using a custom Aquaplast plastic mask with cutouts around the eyes to immobilize the face. After topical anesthesia with proparacaine, a polymethyl methacrylate suction contact lens embedded with a radioopaque wire ring that corresponds to the location of the limbus is placed centered on the cornea. Plain films are used to verify the position of the eye and the head. Figure 2 shows the set-up for a patient with bilateral RB being treated with lateral fields.

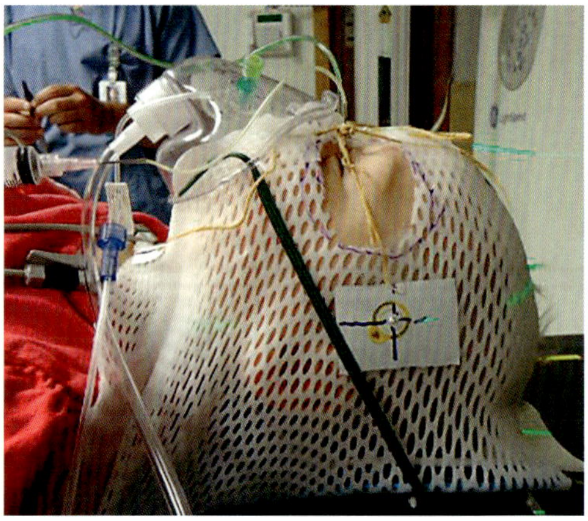

Fig. 2. Patient set-up with custom face immobilization mask (AquaPlast, N.J., USA). A suction contact lens with a radio-opaque wire is used to fix the eyes in a straight-ahead position.

Field Arrangement

Delivering therapeutic dose to the entire retina while minimizing dose to adjacent normal structures is a particular challenge in a region as crowded as the orbit. This is made more difficult by the risk of RT-induced second malignancy in patients with hereditary RB [42]. To minimize this risk, the volume receiving even low dose radiation must be limited as much as possible, as the incidence of sarcomas rises significantly at doses as low as 5 Gy [43].

In 1969, Cassady et al. [13] published the first large series of RB treated with RT. Most patients were treated with a lateral 22.5 MeV Betatron photon field. An anterior field component was avoided to limit both the dose to the brain and anterior segment complications. The anterior edge of the lateral beam was positioned at the lateral bony canthus allowing for quick verification of set-up and treatment without general anesthesia. The relatively poor tumor control of 49% for all eyes, ranging from 84% in RE I to 15% in RE V, was presumed to be from underdosage of the anterior retina and led to the development of combined anterior and lateral beam plans [13].

In 1981, Abramson et al. [15] at Memorial-Sloan Kettering Cancer Center (MSKCC) used the anterior lens-sparing (ALS) approach in which a lateral 10 MeV photon field and anterior 11 MeV electron field were combined and weighted 1:4 (anterior to lateral). The lateral D-shaped (to spare the pituitary and tooth buds) field was blocked anteriorly using a 1 × 1 cm lead shield attached to a contact lens (fig. 3). Although this method appeared to increase dose to the anterior retina, the distribution of dose elsewhere in the retina was less homogenous with the posterior retina being shadowed by the lead shield [15, 16, 21].

In 1996, investigators from MSKCC developed a new technique, the modified lateral beam (MLB), in which a 6 MV lateral D-shaped collimated photon field was positioned 2 mm posterior to the limbus of the eye [16, 21]. The anterior half of the field was blocked (split-beam technique) to sharpen the penumbra. For unilateral disease,

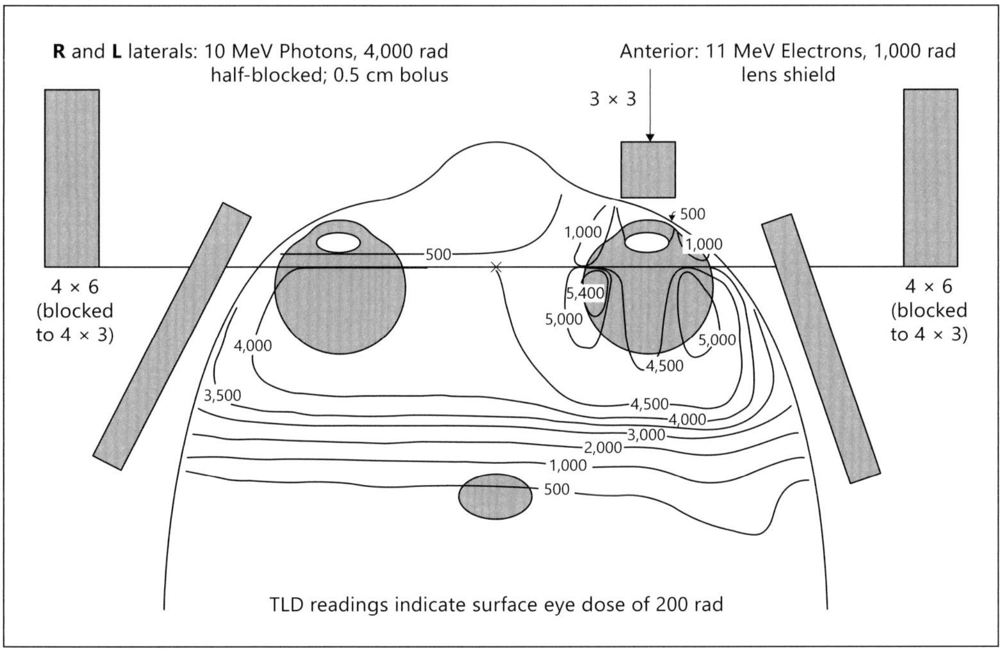

Fig. 3. Anterior lens-sparing approach, which uses a combined anterior and lateral beam with a lead-based lens shield. Reproduced with permission from Abramson et al. [15].

a complex 3-field arrangement was used to minimize dose to contralateral orbit. A superior and inferior 6 MV photon field, each wedged 60° and angled at 90° to each other, delivered the first half to two-thirds of treatment, followed by a lateral 11 MeV electron field that delivered the remaining dose. Blach et al. [21] found that 8-year local control was significantly superior for MLB compared to ALS (65% for MLB vs. 38% for ALS). The rate of ocular survival, however, did not differ significantly (78% for MLB vs. 71% for ALS) [16, 21].

In 1985, Schipper [18] had proposed another lens-sparing lateral beam technique in which the anterior edge of the sharpened beam was positioned tangential to the lens. In cases of anterior tumors or vitreous seeding, the anterior margin was advanced to include 1–3 mm of the posterior lens [19]. An iron rod emerging from the contact lens was magnetically attached to a millimeter scale on the collimator, allowing for a high degree of precision in the placement of the anterior edge of the beam (fig. 4). Unilateral tumors were treated with a single lateral beam obliqued inferiorly to exit through the contralateral maxilla. Ocular salvage at 2 years ranged from 100% in RE I–II to 79% in RE IV [19]. Toma, Hungerford and coworkers compared the Schipper technique to whole eye RT in which the anterior edges of lateral opposed beams were placed a few millimeters anterior to the cornea. The rate of ocular salvage in RE I–III was statistically similar (85% for whole-eye RT vs. 92% for modified Schipper technique), but signifi-

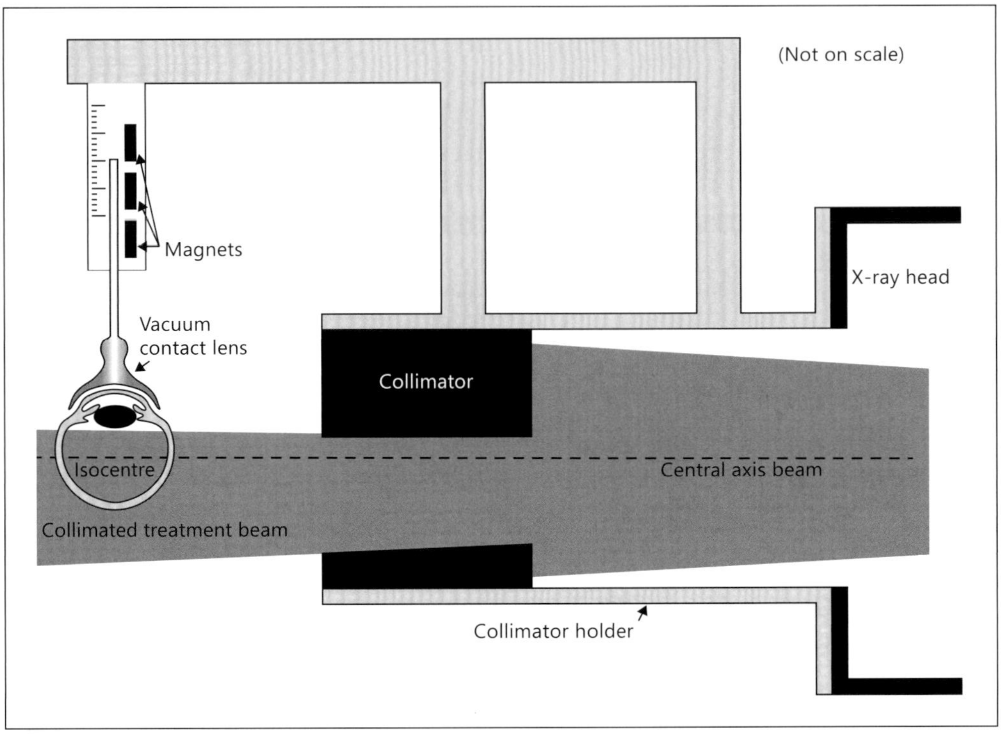

Fig. 4. Lens-sparing lateral beam technique. The contact lens is magnetically coupled to the collimator to allow a high degree of precision in the placement of the anterior edge of the lateral beam. Reproduced with permission from Schipper [18].

cantly fewer anterior recurrences were observed in eyes receiving whole-eye RT [23]. The authors concluded that the modified Schipper technique and other lens-sparing lateral beam strategies provide adequate tumor control and minimal morbidity for eyes belonging to RE I–III. For RE IV–V eyes; however, they recommended whole-eye RT or other techniques that adequately treat the anterior retina [23, 26].

While it is clear that lens-sparing lateral techniques may insufficiently dose the anterior retina, this has not been proven to alter ocular survival, even in advanced RB [44]. Scott et al. [25] compared the relative lens-sparing approach to the MLB. The authors reported a higher rate of local control in RE IV-V disease (81% for relative lens-sparing approach vs. 51% for MLB), but found no significant difference in eye survival, cataract formation or the risk of orbital hypoplasia. Pradhan et al. [17] treated 64 eyes, 67% (43/64) of which were RE IV–V, and found no significant difference in ocular survival between patients treated with a lateral field approach and those treated with a single anterior field or anterior field component. The ability to manage anterior recurrences with laser, cryotherapy or other local therapies may compensate for anterior relapses [16, 21, 30].

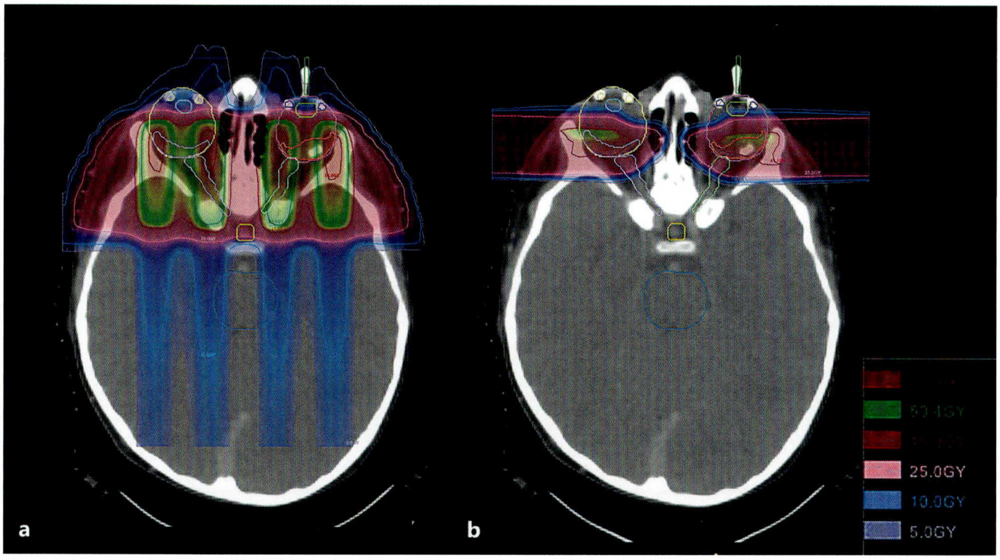

Fig. 5. An anterior and lateral wedged pair photon therapy plan from 1987 used to treat bilateral disease (**a**). Lateral opposed proton therapy plan from 2012 used to treat bilateral disease (**b**). Significantly less low and intermediate dose radiation is delivered to normal tissue.

Nevertheless, many groups have recommended the use of combined anterior and lateral fields for advanced (RE IV–V and ICIR C-D) disease, particularly when the retinal tumor or vitreous seeding extends into the anterior hemisphere [7, 14, 17, 41]. In 1990, Amendola et al. [7] described an anterior and lateral wedged pair without a lens block for RE II–Vb disease. At our institution, before patients began receiving proton RT in 1986, eyes with disease anterior to the equator were treated with a similar technique (fig. 5a). Patients without vitreous seeding and with disease confined to the posterior hemisphere were treated with a technique similar to the MLB.

IMRT may offer significant advantages over conformal photon methods (fig. 6) [44–46]. Krasin et al. [45] compared four techniques: wedged anterior-lateral photon, en face anterior electron field, three-dimensional treatment approach with forward planning, and IMRT. IMRT spared the orbit to a greater degree than any other technique. Reisner et al. [44] comparing 13 techniques found that IMRT adequately treated the ora serrata and the entire vitreous and delivered the second lowest dose to the orbit and the lowest dose to the lacrimal gland. A significant disadvantage of IMRT, however, is the increase in low-dose radiation to normal tissue, a particular concern for RT-induced second malignancy [45].

Proton RT, which our institution has used to treat RB since 1986, may be the ideal form of radiation for RB (fig. 5b). Proton radiation is a form of particle radiation that allows for complete sparing of all structures distal to the target volume and decreased

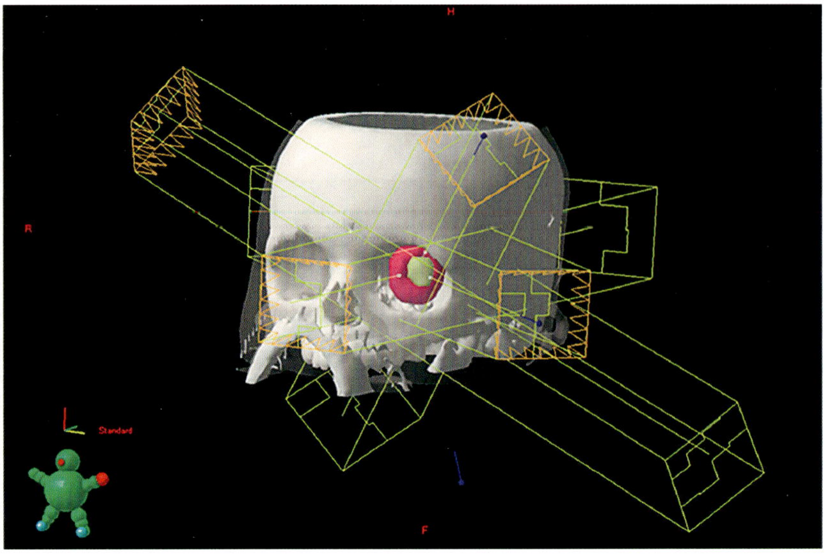

Fig. 6. Four noncoplanar beams used in IMRT treatment of retinoblastoma. Reproduced with permission from Reisner et al. [44].

dose proximal to the target. The use of protons decreases both low and high dose radiation to the surrounding tissues, which should reduce the likelihood of RT-induced second malignancy. In a dosimetric study, Lee et al. [46] compared a single appositional proton beam to IMRT, electron and three-dimensional conformal photons in the treatment of RB. Relative to all other techniques, proton RT provided the best coverage of the retina and delivered the least dose to the bony orbit.

Retinal Capillary Hemangioma

Retinal capillary hemangiomas (RCH) are benign vascular tumors. They are the most common manifestation of von Hippel-Lindau disease, a hereditary cancer syndrome characterized by CNS hemangioblastoma, pheochromocytoma, and renal cell cancer. Maher et al. [47] estimated that RCH are likely to develop in 38% of von Hippel-Lindau disease patients by age 30 years and 70% by age 60 years. Retinal capillary hemangiomas begin as small aneurysmal dilations and progress into a mass of dilated and tortuous vessels [48]. Although benign, RCH poses a serious threat to vision usually by retinal exudation and detachment. The probability of permanent visual loss by the age of 50 is 35% [49]. Most lesions under 4.5 mm can be treated with focal therapy [50, 51]. Although observation is recommended by some for small (≤500 μm), asymptomatic tumors not accompanied by exudation or subretinal fluid, our institution recommends early treatment of small tumors [51, 52].

External Beam Radiation Therapy of Retinal Capillary Hemangioma

Early reports of RCH treated with EBRT found a poor response to treatment [53]. In the last decade, however, there has been renewed interest in the use of RT for large lesions refractory to focal treatments including photocoagulation, cryotherapy, diathermy, and photodynamic therapy. Raja et al. [54] described 6 eyes in 5 patients treated with photons to 21.6 Gy over 12 daily fractions. At a mean follow-up of 28.3 months, the average tumor volume reduction was 27.5 mm^3 or 39.6% of the original volume. Mean visual acuity was 20/70 before treatment and 20/45 after treatment. Small-to-moderate-sized tumors less than 300 mm^3 demonstrated the greatest response to treatment. The major complication was cataract (5/6). The authors recommend EBRT for primary treatment of small-to-moderate RCH that are multifocal, involve the optic disc and/or associated with an exudative retinal detachment.

Palmer and Gragoudas [48] reviewed the outcomes of 10 patients with RCH treated with proton beam RT between 1987 and 1993. The technique was similar to that used to treat choroidal melanomas [55]. A computer model determines the best eye position based on ultrasound measurements of the eye and tumor. Doses between 28 Gy (RBE [relative biological effectiveness]) and 40 Gy (RBE) were prescribed in 4–5 fractions. Additional treatment with photocoagulation and penetrating diathermy was required in 2 patients. Most RCH responded to treatment within 6 months. Five patients had improved or stable vision. Visual acuity in the remaining patients suffered as a result of complications of the underlying tumor. No complications of proton beam RT were reported despite the use of a high fractional dose.

Brachytherapy of Retinal Vascular Tumors

Retinal Capillary Hemangioma

Although widely used in the treatment of choroidal hemangioma, the use of brachytherapy in RCH was not described outside of case reports until 1998 [56, 57]. Kreusel et al. [57] used beta-ray ^{106}Ru and rhodium-106 plaques in the treatment of 25 eyes in 24 patients. The mean scleral contact dose was 518 ± 85 Gy, and the mean apex dose was 126 ± 36 Gy. Dose was delivered over 3–7 days. Twenty-three eyes with RCH exhibited complete regression after a single treatment. In 16 eyes, the visual outcome was favorable (≥20/200 with attached retina). Pretreatment exudative retinal detachment and tumor size larger than 3.75 mm were associated with unfavorable visual outcome. Radiation retinopathy was reported in 1 patient after a second course of brachytherapy. The authors recommend limiting the use of brachytherapy to moderately sized tumors less than 3.75 mm not associated with exudative retinal detachment [57].

Retinal Vasoproliferative Tumor

Larger retinal vasoproliferative tumors can be effectively treated using either ruthenium or iodine plaque brachytherapy [58–61].

Conclusions

The optimal approach to RT of RB is still unknown. In early stage disease, lateral beam approaches (Schipper, MLB) result in adequate ocular salvage and minimize anterior segment morbidity. In patients with vitreous seeding or tumors located anterior to the equator, techniques that increase anterior segment morbidity may be unavoidable. For both early and advanced tumors, highly conformal modalities like proton RT maximize therapeutic dose while minimizing dose to healthy tissue.

Most small RCH and retinal vasoproliferative tumors are treated with photocoagulation and cryotherapy. Larger tumors and/or multifocal lesions refractory to focal therapy may respond to EBRT or brachytherapy.

References

1 Yu CL, Tucker MA, Abramson DH, et al: Cause-specific mortality in long-term survivors of retinoblastoma. J Natl Cancer Inst 2009;101:581–591.

2 Rodriguez-Galindo C, Chantada GL, Haik BG, Wilson MW: Treatment of retinoblastoma: current status and future perspectives. Curr Treat Options Neurol 2007;9:294–307.

3 Reese AB, Ellsworth RM: The evaluation and current concept of retinoblastoma therapy. Trans Am Acad Ophthalmol Otolaryngol 1963;67:164–172.

4 Linn Murphree A: Intraocular retinoblastoma: the case for a new group classification. Ophthalmol Clins N Am 2005;18:41–53, viii.

5 Chantada G, Doz F, Antoneli CB, et al: A proposal for an international retinoblastoma staging system. Pediatr Blood Cancer 2006;47:801–805.

6 Amendola BE, Lamm FR, Markoe AM, et al: Radiotherapy of retinoblastoma. A review of 63 children treated with different irradiation techniques. Cancer 1990;66:21–26.

7 Amendola BE, Markoe AM, Augsburger JJ, et al: Analysis of treatment results in 36 children with retinoblastoma treated by scleral plaque irradiation. Int J Radiat Oncol Biol Phys 1989;17:63–70.

8 Shields CL, Mashayekhi A, Sun H, et al: Iodine-125 plaque radiotherapy as salvage treatment for retinoblastoma recurrence after chemoreduction in 84 tumors. Ophthalmology 2006;113:2087–2092.

9 Shields CL, Shields JA, Cater J, Othmane I, Singh AD, Micaily B: Plaque radiotherapy for retinoblastoma: long-term tumor control and treatment complications in 208 tumors. Ophthalmology 2001;108:2116–2121.

10 Stannard C, Sealy R, Hering E, et al: Localized whole eye radiotherapy for retinoblastoma using a (125)I applicator, 'claws'. Int J Radiat Oncol Biol Phys 2001;51:399–409.

11 Hilgartner H: Report of a case of double glioma treated by X-rays. Tex Med J 1903;18:322–323.

12 Abramson DH, Ellsworth RM, Tretter P, Javitt J, Kitchin FD: Treatment of bilateral groups I through III retinoblastoma with bilateral radiation. Arch Ophthalmol 1981;99:1761–1762.

13 Cassady JR, Sagerman RH, Tretter P, Ellsworth RM: Radiation therapy in retinoblastoma. An analysis of 230 cases. Radiology 1969;93:405–409.

14 Weiss DR, Cassady JR, Petersen R: Retinoblastoma: a modification in radiation therapy technique. Radiology 1975;114:705–708.

15 Abramson DH, Jereb B, Ellsworth RM: External beam radiation for retinoblastoma. Bull NY Acad Med 1981;57:787–803.

16 McCormick B, Ellsworth R, Abramson D, et al: Radiation therapy for retinoblastoma: comparison of results with lens-sparing versus lateral beam techniques. Int J Radiat Oncol Biol Phys 1988;15:567–574.

17 Pradhan DG, Sandridge AL, Mullaney P, et al: Radiation therapy for retinoblastoma: a retrospective review of 120 patients. Int J Radiat Oncol Biol Phys 1997;39:3–13.
18 Schipper J: An accurate and simple method for megavoltage radiation therapy of retinoblastoma. Radiother Oncol 1983;1:31–41.
19 Schipper J, Tan KE, van Peperzeel HA: Treatment of retinoblastoma by precision megavoltage radiation therapy. Radiother Oncol 1985;3:117–132.
20 Abramson DH, Beaverson KL, Chang ST, Dunkel IJ, McCormick B: Outcome following initial external beam radiotherapy in patients with Reese-Ellsworth group Vb retinoblastoma. Arch Ophthalmol 2004; 122:1316–1323.
21 Blach LE, McCormick B, Abramson DH: External beam radiation therapy and retinoblastoma: long-term results in the comparison of two techniques. Int J Radiat Oncol Biol Phys 1996;35:45–51.
22 Hernandez JC, Brady LW, Shields JA, et al: External beam radiation for retinoblastoma: results, patterns of failure, and a proposal for treatment guidelines. Int J Radiat Oncol Biol Phys 1996;35:125–132.
23 Hungerford JL, Toma NM, Plowman PN, Kingston JE: External beam radiotherapy for retinoblastoma. I. Whole eye technique. Br J Ophthalmol 1995;79: 109–111.
24 Merchant TE, Gould CJ, Hilton NE, et al: Ocular preservation after 36 Gy external beam radiation therapy for retinoblastoma. J Pediatr Hematol Oncol 2002;24:246–249.
25 Scott IU, Murray TG, Feuer WJ, et al: External beam radiotherapy in retinoblastoma: tumor control and comparison of 2 techniques. Arch Ophthalmol 1999; 117:766–770.
26 Toma NM, Hungerford JL, Plowman PN, Kingston JE, Doughty D: External beam radiotherapy for retinoblastoma. II. Lens sparing technique. Br J Ophthalmol 1995;79:112–117.
27 Abramson DH, Ellsworth RM, Tretter P, Adams K, Kitchin FD: Simultaneous bilateral radiation for advanced bilateral retinoblastoma. Arch Ophthalmol 1981;99:1763–1766.
28 Imhof SM, Mourits MP, Hofman P, et al: Quantification of orbital and mid-facial growth retardation after megavoltage external beam irradiation in children with retinoblastoma. Ophthalmology 1996;103: 263–268.
29 Shields CL, Honavar SG, Meadows AT, et al: Chemoreduction plus focal therapy for retinoblastoma: factors predictive of need for treatment with external beam radiotherapy or enucleation. Am J Ophthalmol 2002;133:657–664.
30 Abramson DH, Ellsworth RM, Rozakis GW: Cryotherapy for retinoblastoma. Arch Ophthalmol 1982; 100:1253–1256.
31 Turaka K, Shields CL, Meadows AT, Leahey A: Second malignant neoplasms following chemoreduction with carboplatin, etoposide, and vincristine in 245 patients with intraocular retinoblastoma. Pediatr Blood Cancer 2012;59:121–125.
32 Chantada G, Fandino A, Casak S, Manzitti J, Raslawski E, Schvartzman E: Treatment of overt extraocular retinoblastoma. Med Pediatr Oncol 2003;40: 158–161.
33 Chantada G, Fandino A, Davila MT, et al: Results of a prospective study for the treatment of retinoblastoma. Cancer 2004;100:834–842.
34 Antoneli CB, Steinhorst F, de Cassia Braga Ribeiro K, et al: Extraocular retinoblastoma: a 13-year experience. Cancer 2003;98:1292–1298.
35 Rodriguez-Galindo C, Wilson MW, Haik BG, et al: Treatment of metastatic retinoblastoma. Ophthalmology 2003;110:1237–1240.
36 Dunkel IJ, Aledo A, Kernan NA, et al: Successful treatment of metastatic retinoblastoma. Cancer 2000; 89:2117–2121.
37 Kremens B, Wieland R, Reinhard H, et al: High-dose chemotherapy with autologous stem cell rescue in children with retinoblastoma. Bone Marrow Transplant 2003;31:281–284.
38 Blach LE, McCormick B, Abramson DH, Ellsworth RM: Trilateral retinoblastoma – incidence and outcome: a decade of experience. Int J Radiat Oncol Biol Phys 1994;29:729–733.
39 Dunkel IJ, Jubran RF, Gururangan S, et al: Trilateral retinoblastoma: potentially curable with intensive chemotherapy. Pediatr Blood Cancer 2010;54:384–387.
40 Coucke PA, Schmid C, Balmer A, Mirimanoff RO, Thames HD: Hypofractionation in retinoblastoma: an increased risk of retinopathy. Radiother Oncol 1993;28:157–161.
41 Hernandez JC, Brady LW, Shields CL, Shields JA, DePotter P: Conservative treatment of retinoblastoma. The use of plaque brachytherapy. Am J Clin Oncol 1993;16:397–401.
42 Kleinerman RA, Yu CL, Little MP, et al: Variation of second cancer risk by family history of retinoblastoma among long-term survivors. J Clin Oncol 2012; 30:950–957.
43 Wong FL, Boice JD Jr, Abramson DH, et al: Cancer incidence after retinoblastoma. Radiation dose and sarcoma risk. JAMA 1997;278:1262–1267.
44 Reisner ML, Viegas CM, Grazziotin RZ, et al: Retinoblastoma – comparative analysis of external radiotherapy techniques, including an IMRT technique. Int J Radiat Oncol Biol Phys 2007;67:933–941.
45 Krasin MJ, Crawford BT, Zhu Y, et al. Intensity-modulated radiation therapy for children with intraocular retinoblastoma: potential sparing of the bony orbit. Clin Oncol 2004;16:215–222.

46 Lee CT, Bilton SD, Famiglietti RM, et al: Treatment planning with protons for pediatric retinoblastoma, medulloblastoma, and pelvic sarcoma: how do protons compare with other conformal techniques? Int J Radiat Oncol Biol Phys 2005;63:362–372.
47 Maher ER, Yates JR, Harries R, et al: Clinical features and natural history of von Hippel-Lindau disease. Q J Med 1990;77:1151–1163.
48 Palmer JD, Gragoudas ES: Advances in treatment of retinal angiomas. Int Ophthalmol Clin 1997;37:159–170.
49 Webster AR, Maher ER, Moore AT: Clinical characteristics of ocular angiomatosis in von Hippel-Lindau disease and correlation with germline mutation. Arch Ophthalmol 1999;117:371–378.
50 Lane CM, Turner G, Gregor ZJ, Bird AC: Laser treatment of retinal angiomatosis. Eye 1989;3:33–38.
51 Singh AD, Shields CL, Shields JA: von Hippel-Lindau disease. Surv Ophthalmol 2001;46:117–142.
52 Singh AD, Nouri M, Shields CL, Shields JA, Perez N: Treatment of retinal capillary hemangioma. Ophthalmology 2002;109:1799–1806.
53 Ballantyne AJ: Angiomatosis retinae. Account of a case, including the histological results of X-ray treatment. Proc R Soc Med 1942;35:345–358.
54 Raja D, Benz MS, Murray TG, Escalona-Benz EM, Markoe A: Salvage external beam radiotherapy of retinal capillary hemangiomas secondary to von Hippel-Lindau disease: visual and anatomic outcomes. Ophthalmology 2004;111:150–153.
55 Gragoudas ES, Goitein M, Verhey L, Munzenreider J, Suit HD, Koehler A: Proton beam irradiation. An alternative to enucleation for intraocular melanomas. Ophthalmology 1980;87:571–581.
56 Balazs E, Berta A, Rozsa L, Kolozsvari L, Rigo G: Hemodynamic changes after ruthenium irradiation of Hippel's angiomatosis. Ophthalmologica 1990;200:128–132.
57 Kreusel KM, Bornfeld N, Lommatzsch A, Wessing A, Foerster MH: Ruthenium-106 brachytherapy for peripheral retinal capillary hemangioma. Ophthalmology 1998;105:1386–1392.
58 Shields CL, Shields JA, Barrett J, De Potter P: Vasoproliferative tumors of the ocular fundus. Classification and clinical manifestations in 103 patients. Arch Ophthalmol 1995;113:615–623.
59 Heimann H, Bornfeld N, Vij O, et al: Vasoproliferative tumours of the retina. Br J Ophthalmol 2000;84:1162–1169.
60 Cohen VML, Shields CL, Demirci H, Shields JA: Iodine I 125 plaque radiotherapy for vasoproliferative tumors of the retina in 30 eyes. Arch Ophthalmol 2008;126:1245–1251.
61 Anastassiou G, Bornfeld N, Schueler AO, et al: Ruthenium-106 plaque brachytherapy for symptomatic vasoproliferative tumours of the retina (comment). Br J Ophthalmol 2006;90:447–450.

Shizuo Mukai, MD
Retina Service, Massachusetts Eye and Ear Infirmary
243 Charles Street
Boston, MA 02114 (USA)
E-Mail Shizuo_Mukai@meei.harvard.edu

Singh AD, Pelayes DE, Seregard S, Macklis R (eds): Ophthalmic Radiation Therapy. Techniques and Applications.
Dev Ophthalmol. Basel, Karger, 2013, vol 52, pp 75–84 (DOI: 10.1159/000351061)

Radiation Therapy: Age-Related Macular Degeneration

Carlos A. Medina Mendez · Justis P. Ehlers
Vitreoretinal Service, Cleveland Clinic Cole Eye Institute, Cleveland, Ohio, USA

Abstract
Age-related macular degeneration (AMD) is the leading cause of severe irreversible vision loss in patients over the age of 50 years in the developed world. Neovascular AMD (NVAMD) is responsible for 90% of the cases with severe visual loss. In the last decade, the treatment paradigm for NVAMD has been transformed by the advent of anti-vascular endothelial growth factor therapy. Despite the excellent results of anti-vascular endothelial growth factor therapy, frequent injections remain a necessity for most patients. The burden of these frequent visits as well as the cumulative risks of indefinite intravitreal injections demand continued pursuit of more enduring therapy that provides similar functional results. Radiotherapy has been studied for two decades as a potential therapy for NVAMD. Because of its antiangiogenic properties, radiation therapy remains a promising potential adjunctive resource for the treatment of choroidal neovascularization secondary to NVAMD. This review considers the past, present and future of radiation as a treatment or combination treatment of NVAMD.

Age-related macular degeneration (AMD) is the leading cause of severe, irreversible visual loss in patients over the age of 50 years in the developed world, including the United States and United Kingdom [1–4]. The prevalence of this disease has been increasing as life expectancy continues to increase [4]. In the United States, an estimated 1.75 million people suffer from advanced AMD, a number predicted to rise to near 3 million by the year 2020 [4].

The hallmark of AMD is drusen, which are yellow subretinal deposits that are often accompanied by hypo- or hyperpigmentary changes of the retinal pigment epithelium. AMD has been grossly stratified as either non-neovascular/atrophic (dry) or neovascular/exudative (wet). Although neovascular AMD (NVAMD) represents only 10–15% of the cases, it is responsible for 90% of the cases with severe visual loss [5]. Typical symptoms include decreased central vision, central scotoma and metamorphopsia.

Development and progression of choroidal neovascularization (CNV) is the hallmark of NVAMD. CNV occurs when abnormal blood vessels develop in the subretinal pigment epithelium (RPE) or subretinal space. It is believed that oxidative stress to the RPE leads to the formation of drusen from the accumulation of extracellular debris. Drusen alter the permeability of Bruch's membrane to nutrients and damage the integrity of Bruch's membrane, which may eventually lead to RPE atrophy or CNV development [6, 7]. Extracellular deposition of diffuse basal laminar drusen and linear deposits between the cytoplasmic and basement membrane of the RPE are significantly associated with CNV formation [8, 9]. Visual loss from NVAMD occurs when CNV activity results in hemorrhage or leakage of fluid into or under the retina and/or RPE [10]. If left untreated, gliosis/fibrosis occurs leading to severe vision loss and a disciform scar characteristic of end-stage NVAMD.

Although much remains elusive about the etiology of AMD, it is clear that genetics and the inflammatory pathway are involved in the pathogenesis of AMD. The greatest risk factor for AMD is age, with individuals over 50 years of age having greater risk compared to those under 50 [11, 12]. Cigarette smoking is the most important modifiable frisk factor associated with AMD [13]. Other modifiable risk factors include body mass index, hypertension, cardiovascular disease and alcohol consumption [14]. Whether or not exposure to sunlight increases the risk of AMD is still controversial [15, 16].

CNV is the leading cause of AMD-related visual loss [17]. Significant advances in the understanding of CNV pathogenesis have led to several FDA-approved therapies for NVAMD. Laser photocoagulation was one of the first therapies advocated for NVAMD. However, the results of laser photocoagulation were disappointing. Laser photocoagulation induced full thickness retinal burns and immediate loss of visual acuity with a 50% recurrence rate, especially with subfoveal neovascularization [18]. Other therapies including subretinal surgery and macular translocation have also been explored with variable success [19–22]. Photodynamic therapy was initially thought to be a major breakthrough for the treatment of NVAMD. Although it was successful in reducing the loss of 3 lines of vision, very few eyes gained any vision. Unfortunately, few patients gained vision with photodynamic therapy [23, 24].

In the last decade, the treatment paradigm for NVAMD has been transformed by the advent of anti-vascular endothelial growth factor (VEGF) therapy [25–31]. Multicenter, randomized, controlled studies have showed that sustained treatment with intravitreal injections of anti-VEGF therapy (e.g. bevacizumab, ranibizumab, aflibercept) are effective in not only reducing the loss of vision but improving visual function in many patients with neovascular AMD [25–31]. Despite the excellent results of anti-VEGF therapy, frequent injections remain a necessity for most patients. The burden of these frequent visits as well as the cumulative risks of indefinite intravitreal injections demand continued pursuit of more enduring therapy that provides similar functional results.

Principles of Radiation Treatment for Age-Related Macular Degeneration

Radiotherapy has been studied for two decades as a potential therapy for NVAMD with data on radiation as a treatment for choroidal neovascularization first reported in the literature in 1993 [32]. The concept of radiation for the treatment of NVAMD is based on the notion that radiation primarily affects proliferating cells by causing free radicals with irreparable damage to DNA and protein synthesis limiting CNV proliferation. It is thought that CNV pathophysiology is similar to that of proliferative wound healing. Theoretically, the proliferating cells within the CNV complex would be more sensitive to radiation and be affected at doses that would not significantly damage the surrounding nonproliferating cells of the retina [33]. Although the cells in the surrounding area are exposed to the radiation, these nondividing cells are able to repair the damaged DNA whereas, the rapidly proliferating cells within the CNV either discontinue cell division or undergo apoptosis [34, 35].

In general, radiation used for medical therapies can be divided into two main categories depending on the method of delivery. External beam radiation or teletherapy uses radiation from an isotope or an electromagnetic source, which is formed into a beam that is projected to a targeted internal body tissue from that external source [33, 36]. Brachytherapy uses a radiation source delivered directly over the tissue almost always requiring surgery. The source is usually an isotope that produces ionizing radiation as it decays and emits energy.

External Beam Radiation

External beam radiation was the first type of radiation to be studied for the treatment of NVAMD. The use of external beam radiation carries a major disadvantage as the high-energy radiation must penetrate through the ocular and periocular tissue and to target the CNV at the macula. This can cause significant collateral side effects. Several studies have shown isolated external beam radiotherapy results to be better than the natural history of the disease but these results do not match the outstanding results of the anti-VEGF era [25–31, 37, 38]. External beam radiation was developed to target tumor lesions that are typically much larger in size than CNV. Therefore, targeting CNV is difficult with standard external beam radiation without getting significant collateral damage to ocular and periocular tissues.

Stereotactic Radiotherapy

Recently, stereotactic radiotherapy or radiosurgery has been studied for the treatment of CNV. This treatment directs beams from different angles targeting radiation onto the target tissue and minimizing exposure to the surrounding tissue. The system is designed to divide the dose into several separate beams that will cause less collateral damage to the surrounding tissue while focusing the full dose treatment to the area of interest. The IRay™ is a robotic stereotactic radiotherapy platform designed to operate in the ophthalmologist's office using a 220–240 V wall socket and without the need

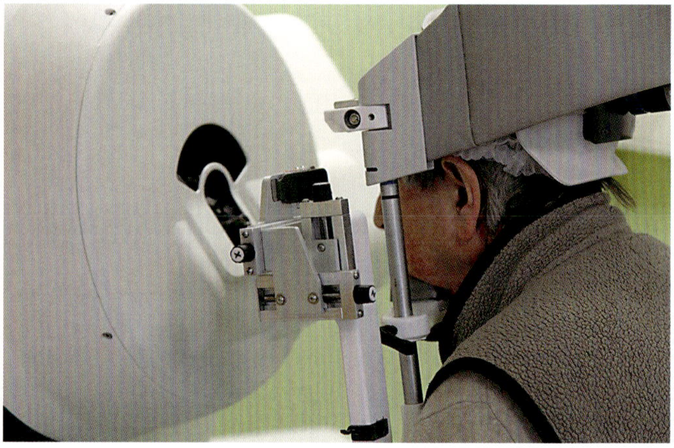

Fig. 1. I-Ray system that uses a coupling device with suction to fixate the eye and direct radiotherapy through the pars plana and into the macula while avoiding the lens.

for room shielding. It is designed to deliver radiation to the macula via three separate locations through the inferior pars plana (fig. 1). The radiation source uses a robotically controlled delivery system connected to the patient using a vacuum-coupled contact lens. The system can track eye movements and redirect treatment and or stop treatment if the eye moves out of position. Currently, the IRay system is under investigation for the treatment of NVAMD [39].

Brachytherapy

Currently, plaque brachytherapy and epimacular brachytherapy are being studied. Plaque brachytherapy has the advantage that the plaque is sutured directly onto the sclera posterior to the macula and therefore the target tissue dosage variability is greatly reduced when compared to other delivery methods. This also means that plaques are usually aimed towards the lens, the most radiosensitive structure in the eye often producing radiation related cataracts. Plaque brachytherapy also requires at least two surgical procedures, one to insert and a second to remove the plaque.

Epimacular brachytherapy was developed to deliver targeted intrasurgical intraocular targeted radiation. Radiation is delivered following pars plana vitrectomy. Once the vitreous has been removed the surgeon positions a probe over the CNV lesion for a short period of time (e.g. less than 5 min). Because of the exponential decrease in radiation exposure with increasing distance from the radiation source the radiation dose to adjacent tissue is low. In addition to the radiation therapy, vitrectomy alone may have some beneficial effect on NVAMD progression due to increased oxygen availability in the vitreous cavity [33, 40, 41]. Increased oxygen concentration in the vitreous is thought to have a positive effect and decrease the progression of macular degeneration. Disadvantages of epimacular brachytherapy are that it requires complex surgery as well as the introduction of surgeon error/variability in dosing as the probe can be placed at different distances to the targeted tissue.

Combination Therapy

There are several theoretical advantages for the use of combined anti-VEGF and radiotherapy for NVAMD. Unlike current anti-VEGF therapies, radiation therapy could provide a more durable effect. Current success with anti-VEGF therapies have set new standards to which all new AMD therapies must be evaluated. New and/or combined treatments must either have significantly improved efficacy, a longer-lasting effect or a safer and more convenient mode of delivery. Combination therapies must be evaluated and considered according to these criteria [42]. VEGF targeting agents have a rapid onset of action but limited durability in many patients, as disease tends to recur if treatment is withheld [25–31]. On the other hand, radiation effects on CNV often require months to take full effect [33]. It can be hypothesized that the two therapies may have an additive if not synergistic effect when combined [33]. Combination therapy with anti-VEGF agents and radiotherapy are being widely pursued as combination treatment of oncologic disease such as colon cancer [43]. As the VEGF targeting agents inhibit growth factors, radiotherapy disables the local inflammatory response and vascular endothelial cell proliferation. The potential benefits of these two approaches could result in a more durable and possibly more complete recovery of vision.

Clinical Studies of Radiation Therapy for NVAMD

External Beam Radiation

Randomized control trials utilizing radiotherapy alone have thus far been associated with only a modest benefit for the treatment of AMD [44]. External beam radiation has been the primary mode of experimental radiation therapy for AMD. To date, there are 13 randomized clinical trials investigating the efficacy of external beam radiotherapy with does ranging from 7.5 to 24 Gy. Data analyzed in a recent Cochrane database review [38] reveals most studies found effects that favored the radiation therapy although these where not always statistically significant and these marginal results must be considered in context of the anti-VEGF era. Many of these trials have major limitations including the lack of double masking and because of this were considered to be at risk of bias [38, 45, 46].

Recently, external beam radiation has been revised and stereotactic radiotherapy or radiosurgery has been studied for the treatment of NVAMD. Combination therapy utilizing anti-VEGF and the previously described IRay system, which uses a low-voltage X-ray source, is now being studied. The IRay may be used in the office setting to pass three beams of radiation through the inferior pars plana and into the macula. CLH001 was a single-center uncontrolled pilot study that included 62 patients who had already received anti-VEGF and others who were treatment naïve. Subjects received either 16 or 24 Gy and different induction regimens. Induction regimens included anti-VEGF therapy at baseline and month 1 with radiotherapy in between or radiotherapy only at baseline. Anti-VEGF was then administered as required based on disease activity. At 12 months visual acuity had stabilized or improved for the majority of patients. The mean gain has been 8–10 ETDRS letters and there were no device-related serious adverse effects (12-month data were presented by Peter Kaiser at Angiogenesis Feb. 20, 2010 and again by Darius Moshfeghi at Macula Society Feb. 24–27, 2010) [33]. CLH002 or INTREPID (Iray Plus Anti-VEGF Treatment for Patients with Wet AMD) is a phase II multinational, randomized controlled study evaluating the safety and establish the effectiveness of two doses from the IRay System for the treatment of wet AMD in patients who have already been treated with anti-VEGF therapy. The trial included 230 patients that received at least three anti-VEGF injections in the year prior to recruitment and required ongoing anti-VEGF treatment. Within 2 weeks after injection, one third of patients received a sham exposure, one third received a radiation dose of either 16 Gy, and one third received 24 Gy. Patients were followed monthly and treated with ranibizumab as needed. A statistically significant reduction of approximately 35% injections was seen in the treated versus the sham group with similar or improved visual acuity outcomes. The number of adverse events and serious adverse events were similar across arms and no radiation related adverse effects occurred at the 1-year endpoint [46, 47]. The IRay system is now available commercially in the UK, and soon in Switzerland and other European countries.

Brachytherapy

Radioactive plaque brachytherapy has also been extensively studied. Palladium-103 was the first isotope to be used in the treatment of NVAMD [48]. In 1999, Finger and colleagues published their nonrandomized phase I study where they reported 23 patients who underwent brachytherapy treatment for NVAMD with doses of 12.5 to 23.6 Gy to the retina apex. Two-year follow-up showed an 87% rate of stable or improved fundoscopic and angiographic findings though 1/3 of the patients developed recurrent lesions [48]. Long-term follow-up published a reported visual acuity at 33.3 months is as follows: improvement of ≥3 ETDRS lines in 16% of patients, loss of ≥3 ETDRS lines in 55% of patients. The remaining 29% of patients remained within 2 ETDRS lines of visual acuity from baseline [49]. Results do not fare well when compared to anti-VEGF therapy.

Epimacular brachytherapy using the Epi-rad strontium-90 source have also been studied (Neovista). As previously discussed Epi-rad uses an endoscopic probe to deliver radiation over the lesion. In one study, patients undergo a 3-port pars plana vitrectomy after which the probe is held in apposition to the retinal surface for less than 5 min to deliver the dose of 24 Gy. Patients also receive an intravitreal injection of anti-VEGF therapy. Thirty-four patients were included in this open label, non-controlled, non-randomized, multicenter, prospective phase I clinical trial. These treatment naïve subjects received either 15 Gy (4 patients) or 24 Gy (17 patients) of beta irradiation [50]. Thirty-four subjects were followed-up for 24 months and 19 were followed-up through 36 months. Mean best-corrected visual acuity demonstrated an average gain of +15.0 and –4.9 letters at 12 and 24 months, respectively. The drop in mean gain at month 24 was largely attributable to cataract formation. At 36 months 90% of eyes had lost <15 letters from baseline, 53% of eyes had gain ≥1 letter while 21% of eyes had gained ≥15 letters. Through 36 months, 11 eyes required additional bevacizumab retreatment therapy and received a mean of 3.0 injections (range 2–7 injections) [50]. This device was evaluated in two prospective, randomized, controlled trials in treatment-naive subjects (CABERNET) and in subjects already treated with anti-VEGF therapy (MERLOT). CABERNET included 457 previously treatment naïve patients with all types of NVAMD. Patients were randomized into 302 patients in the treatment arm and 155 patients in the control arm. At 2 years 77% of the radiation-treated group and 90% of the control group lost fewer than 15 ETDRS letters from baseline. The difference did not achieve its prespecified 10% noninferiority margin. Results showed that the epimacular brachytherapy treatment group required a mean of 6.2 injections at 2 years for a mean visual acuity loss of 2.5 letters while the control group receiving ranibizumab monotherapy required a mean of 10.4 injections at 2 years to achieve a mean gain of 4.4 letters. The 2-year efficacy data did not support the routine use of epimacular brachytherapy for the treatment of naïve wet AMD [51, 52].

Safety

Delivery of external beam radiation is not localized and collateral damage to healthy tissue is inevitable. Long-term follow-up is needed as radiation toxicity can occur up to 15 years after treatment [53, 54]. The crystalline lens is exquisitely sensitive to radiation and doses of less than 2 Gy have been reported to cause cataracts [55]. The formation of cataracts may occur as early as 1 month following treatment and as late as 7 years depending upon several factors including the type of radiation, total dose, delivery portals and the time after exposure [56]. Radiation has been primarily associated with posterior subcapsular cataracts.

Because the neural elements of the retina are relatively resistant to radiation, the destructive effects of radiation are largely mediated through damage to the retinal vasculature where vascular changes show a progressive pattern of capillary closure, dilation and leakage [57]. The effect is proportional to the dose, fraction size and duration of treatment as well as coexisting comorbidities, such as diabetes mellitus. Absolute figures regarding a safe dose are still unknown; however, clinical and experimental data suggest that doses under 2,500 cGy in fractions of 200 cGy or less are unlikely to cause significant retinopathy [58]. As previously discussed, brachytherapy would provide more direct dosing to the tissue of interest but usually requires a surgical procedure that itself carries safety concerns such as infection, scleral perforation, and the risk of anesthesia.

Conclusion

Because of its anti-angiogenic properties, radiation therapy remains a promising potential adjunctive resource for the treatment of NVAMD [57, 59, 60]. Currently, there are no FDA-approved therapies utilizing radiation for the treatment of NVAMD. Multiple clinical trials are ongoing including both brachytherapy devices and novel stereotactic radiotherapy devices. Long-term safety concerns still exist as late effects from radiation may be seen even years after initial exposure, and the definitive benefit to anti-VEGF monotherapy (whether in endurance or magnitude of effect) remains unclear at this time. The future of radiotherapy in NVAMD depends on the development of new devices to deliver radiation in a safe, reproducible and cost-effective manner that reduces patient/physician visit burden and improves/maintains current visual outcomes. Certain patients or disease phenotypes may be particularly amenable to radiotherapy and/or combination therapy, including patients with incomplete or short-lived response to current treatments.

References

1 Brown MM, Brown GC, Sharma S, Stein JD, Roth Z, Campanella J, et al: The burden of age-related macular degeneration: a value-based analysis. Curr Opin Ophthalmol 2006;17:257–266.

2 Evans JR, Fletcher AE, Wormald RP: Causes of visual impairment in people aged 75 years and older in Britain: an add-on study to the MRC Trial of Assessment and Management of Older People in the Community. Br J Ophthalmol 2004;88:365–370.

3 Klein R, Klein BE, Tomany SC, Meuer SM, Huang GH: Ten-year incidence and progression of age-related maculopathy: the Beaver Dam eye study. Ophthalmology 2002;109:1767–1779.

4 Friedman DS, O'Colmain BJ, Munoz B, Tomany SC, McCarty C, de Jong PT, et al: Prevalence of age-related macular degeneration in the United States. Arch Ophthalmol 2004;122:564–572.

5 Ferris FL 3rd, Fine SL, Hyman L: Age-related macular degeneration and blindness due to neovascular maculopathy. Arch Ophthalmol 1984;102:1640–1642.

6 Zarbin MA: Age-related macular degeneration: review of pathogenesis. Eur J Ophthalmol 1998;8:199–206.

7 Beatty S, Koh H, Phil M, Henson D, Boulton M: The role of oxidative stress in the pathogenesis of age-related macular degeneration. Surv Ophthalmol 2000; 45:115–134.

8 Grossniklaus HE, Green WR: Histopathologic and ultrastructural findings of surgically excised choroidal neovascularization. Submacular Surgery Trials Research Group. Arch Ophthalmol 1998;116:745–749.

9 Lopez PF, Grossniklaus HE, Lambert HM, Aaberg TM, Capone A Jr, Sternberg P Jr, et al: Pathologic features of surgically excised subretinal neovascular membranes in age-related macular degeneration. Am J Ophthalmol 1991;112:647–656.

10 Yuan A, Kaiser PK: Emerging therapies for the treatment of neovascular age related macular degeneration. Semin Ophthalmol 2011;26:149–155.

11 Friedman DS, Katz J, Bressler NM, Rahmani B, Tielsch JM: Racial differences in the prevalence of age-related macular degeneration: the Baltimore Eye Survey. Ophthalmology 1999;106:1049–1055.

12 VanNewkirk MR, Nanjan MB, Wang JJ, Mitchell P, Taylor HR, McCarty CA: The prevalence of age-related maculopathy: the visual impairment project. Ophthalmology 2000;107:1593–1600.

13 Thornton J, Edwards R, Mitchell P, Harrison RA, Buchan I, Kelly SP: Smoking and age-related macular degeneration: a review of association. Eye (Lond) 2005;19:935–944.

14 Klein R: Overview of progress in the epidemiology of age-related macular degeneration. Ophthalmic Epidemiol 2007;14:184–187.

15 Cruickshanks KJ, Klein R, Klein BE, Nondahl DM: Sunlight and the 5-year incidence of early age-related maculopathy: the Beaver Dam Eye Study. Arch Ophthalmol 2001;119:246–250.

16 Delcourt C, Carriere I, Ponton-Sanchez A, Fourrey S, Lacroux A, Papoz L: Light exposure and the risk of age-related macular degeneration: the Pathologies Oculaires Liees a l'Age (POLA) study. Arch Ophthalmol 2001;119:1463–1468.

17 Couch SM, Bakri SJ: Review of combination therapies for neovascular age-related macular degeneration. Semin Ophthalmol 2011;26:114–120.
18 Macular Photocoagulation Study Group: Argon laser photocoagulation for neovascular maculopathy. Five-year results from randomized clinical trials. Arch Ophthalmol 1991;109:1109–1114.
19 Hawkins BS, Bressler NM, Miskala PH, Bressler SB, Holekamp NM, Marsh MJ, et al: Surgery for subfoveal choroidal neovascularization in age-related macular degeneration: ophthalmic findings. SST report No. 11. Ophthalmology 2004;111:1967–1980.
20 Bressler NM, Bressler SB, Childs AL, Haller JA, Hawkins BS, Lewis H, et al: Surgery for hemorrhagic choroidal neovascular lesions of age-related macular degeneration: ophthalmic findings. SST report No. 13. Ophthalmology 2004;111:1993–2006.
21 Chen FK, Patel PJ, Uppal GS, Tufail A, Coffey PJ, Da Cruz L: Long-term outcomes following full macular translocation surgery in neovascular age-related macular degeneration. Br J Ophthalmol 2010;94:1337–1343.
22 Eandi CM, Giansanti F, Virgili G: Macular translocation for neovascular age-related macular degeneration. Cochrane Database Syst Rev 2008;4:CD006928.
23 Photodynamic therapy of subfoveal choroidal neovascularization in age-related macular degeneration with verteporfin: one-year results of 2 randomized clinical trials – TAP report. Treatment of Age-Related Macular Degeneration with Photodynamic Therapy (TAP) Study Group. Arch Ophthalmol 1999; 117:1329–1345.
24 Verteporfin therapy of subfoveal choroidal neovascularization in age-related macular degeneration: two-year results of a randomized clinical trial including lesions with occult with no classic choroidal neovascularization – verteporfin in photodynamic therapy report 2. Am J Ophthalmol 2001;131:541–560.
25 Brown DM, Kaiser PK, Michels M, Soubrane G, Heier JS, Kim RY, et al: Ranibizumab versus verteporfin for neovascular age-related macular degeneration. N Engl J Med 2006;355:1432–1444.
26 Colquitt JL, Jones J, Tan SC, Takeda A, Clegg AJ, Price A: Ranibizumab and pegaptanib for the treatment of age-related macular degeneration: a systematic review and economic evaluation. Health Technol Assess 2008;12:iii–iv, ix–201.
27 Rosenfeld PJ, Brown DM, Heier JS, Boyer DS, Kaiser PK, Chung CY, et al: Ranibizumab for neovascular age-related macular degeneration. N Engl J Med 2006;355:1419–1431.
28 Nguyen QD, Heier J, Brown D, Ho A, Kaiser P, Vitti R, et al: Randomized, double-masked, active-controlled phase 3 trial of the efficacy and safety of intravitreal VEGF trap-eye in wet AMD: one-year results of the VIew-1 study IOVS. ARVO 2011, abstr 3073.
29 Chakravarthy U, Harding SP, Rogers CA, Downes SM, Lotery AJ, Wordsworth S, et al: Ranibizumab versus bevacizumab to treat neovascular age-related macular degeneration: one-year findings from the IVAN randomized trial. Ophthalmology 2012;119: 1399–1411.
30 Martin DF, Maguire MG, Ying GS, Grunwald JE, Fine SL, Jaffe GJ: Ranibizumab and bevacizumab for neovascular age-related macular degeneration. N Engl J Med 2011;364:1897–1908.
31 Heier JS, Brown DM, Chong V, Korobelnik JF, Kaiser PK, Nguyen QD, et al: Intravitreal Aflibercept (VEGF Trap-Eye) in wet age-related macular degeneration. Ophthalmology 2012;119:2537–2548.
32 Chakravarthy U, Houston RF, Archer DB: Treatment of age-related subfoveal neovascular membranes by teletherapy: a pilot study. Br J Ophthalmol 1993;77:265–273.
33 Petrarca R, Jackson TL: Radiation therapy for neovascular age-related macular degeneration. Clin Ophthalmol 2011;5:57–63.
34 Kirwan JF, Constable PH, Murdoch IE, Khaw PT: Beta irradiation: new uses for an old treatment: a review. Eye (Lond) 2003;17:207–215.
35 Trikha R, Morse LS, Zawadzki RJ, Werner JS, Park SS: Ten-year follow-up of eyes treated with stereotactic fractionated external beam radiation for neovascular age-related macular degeneration. Retina 2011;31:1303–1315.
36 Barnhard HJ: Supervoltage therapy comes of age: a report for the practicing physician. N Engl J Med 1958;258:275–277.
37 Chakravarthy U, MacKenzie G: External beam radiotherapy in exudative age-related macular degeneration: a pooled analysis of phase I data. Br J Radiol 2000;73:305–313.
38 Evans JR, Sivagnanavel V, Chong V: Radiotherapy for neovascular age-related macular degeneration. Cochrane Database Syst Rev 2010;5:CD004004.
39 Moshfeghi DM, Kaiser PK, Gertner M: Stereotactic low-voltage X-ray irradiation for age-related macular degeneration. Br J Ophthalmol 2011;95:185–188.
40 Jampol LM: Oxygen therapy and intraocular oxygenation. Trans Am Ophthalmol Soc 1987;85:407–437.
41 Stefansson E, Landers MB 3rd, Wolbarsht ML: Increased retinal oxygen supply following pan-retinal photocoagulation and vitrectomy and lensectomy. Trans Am Ophthalmol Soc 1981;79:307–334.
42 Kim IK, Gragoudas ES: Radiation therapy for neovascular age-related macular degeneration revisited. Br J Ophthalmol 2009;93:279–280.
43 Senan S, Smit EF: Design of clinical trials of radiation combined with antiangiogenic therapy. Oncologist 2007;12:465–477.
44 Sivagnanavel V, Evans JR, Ockrim Z, Chong V: Radiotherapy for neovascular age-related macular degeneration. Cochrane Database Syst Rev 2004;4:CD004004.

45 Silva RA, Moshfeghi AA, Kaiser PK, Singh RP, Moshfeghi DM: Radiation treatment for age-related macular degeneration. Semin Ophthalmol 2011;26: 121–130.
46 Jackson TL, Chakravarthy U, Kaiser PK, Slakter JS, Jan E, Bandello F, et al: Stereotactic Radiotherapy for Neovascular Age-Related Macular Degeneration: 52-Week Safety and Efficacy Results of the INTREPID Study. Ophthalmology, in press.
47 Jackson TL: INTREPID data and its significance. 12th Euretina Congress, Milan, 2012.
48 Finger PT, Berson A, Sherr D, Riley R, Balkin RA, Bosworth JL: Radiation therapy for subretinal neovascularization. Ophthalmology 1996;103:878–889.
49 Finger PT, Berson A, Ng T, Szechter A: Ophthalmic plaque radiotherapy for age-related macular degeneration associated with subretinal neovascularization. Am J Ophthalmol 1999;127:170–177.
50 Avila MP, Farah ME, Santos A, Carla L, Fuji G, Rossi J, et al: Three-year safety and visual acuity results of epimacular 90 strontium/90 yttrium brachytherapy with bevacizumab for the treatment of subfoveal choroidal neovascularization secondary to age-related macular degeneration. Retina 2012;32:10–18.
51 Dugel P: CABERNET: for treatment of naive neovascular macular degeneration. Angiogenesis, Miami, 2012.
52 Dugel PU, Bebchuk JD, Nau J, Reichel E, Singer M, Barak A, et al: Epimacular brachytherapy for neovascular age-related macular degeneration: a randomized, controlled trial (CABERNET). Ophthalmology 2013;120:317–327.
53 Guyer DR, Mukai S, Egan KM, Seddon JM, Walsh SM, Gragoudas ES: Radiation maculopathy after proton beam irradiation for choroidal melanoma. Ophthalmology 1992;99:1278–1285.
54 Flaxel CJ: Use of radiation in the treatment of age-related macular degeneration. Ophthalmol Clin North Am 2002;15:437–444, v.
55 Hoehn ME, Irshad F, Kerr NC, Wilson MW: Outcomes after cataract extraction in young children with radiation-induced cataracts and retinoblastoma. J AAPOS 2010;14:232–234.
56 Cogan DG, Donaldson DD, Reese AB: Clinical and pathological characteristics of radiation cataract. AMA Arch Ophthalmol 1952;47:55–70.
57 Archer DB, Gardiner TA: Ionizing radiation and the retina. Curr Opin Ophthalmol 1994;5:59–65.
58 Archer DB: Doyne Lecture. Responses of retinal and choroidal vessels to ionising radiation. Eye (Lond) 1993;7:1–13.
59 Rodel F, Keilholz L, Herrmann M, Sauer R, Hildebrandt G: Radiobiological mechanisms in inflammatory diseases of low-dose radiation therapy. Int J Radiat Biol 2007;83:357–366.
60 Wachsberger P, Burd R, Dicker AP: Tumor response to ionizing radiation combined with antiangiogenesis or vascular targeting agents: exploring mechanisms of interaction. Clin Cancer Res 2003;9:1957–1971.

Justis P. Ehlers, MD
Vitreoretinal Service, Cleveland Clinic Cole Eye Institute
9500 Euclid Avenue, Mail Code i-32
Cleveland, OH 44195 (USA)
E-Mail ehlersj@ccf.org

Singh AD, Pelayes DE, Seregard S, Macklis R (eds): Ophthalmic Radiation Therapy. Techniques and Applications.
Dev Ophthalmol. Basel, Karger, 2013, vol 52, pp 85–93 (DOI: 10.1159/000351062)

Radiation Therapy: Conjunctival and Eyelid Tumors

Mary E. Aronow · Arun D. Singh

Department of Ophthalmic Oncology, Cole Eye Institute, Cleveland Clinic Foundation, Cleveland, Ohio, USA

Abstract

While the primary treatment of eyelid and conjunctival tumors is frequently surgical, several forms of ophthalmic radiation therapy have also been used to treat these malignancies. The goal of radiation therapy is to eradicate tumor burden in a manner that maintains visual function and preserves surrounding sensitive ocular tissues. Ophthalmic radiation may be used as a curative therapy, as adjuvant treatment following surgical excision, or as palliative therapy for advanced cases of eyelid and conjunctival tumors. The following review discusses the indications and outcomes of various modalities of radiation (external beam radiotherapy and brachytherapy) used to treat eyelid tumors (squamous cell carcinoma, basal cell carcinoma, sebaceous gland carcinoma, and melanoma) and conjunctival tumors (squamous cell carcinoma and melanoma).

Ophthalmic radiation therapy in several forms has been used with success to treat eyelid and conjunctival malignancies. As with other ocular tumors, the goal of radiation therapy is to eradicate tumor burden in a manner that maintains visual function and preserves surrounding sensitive ocular tissues. In the following chapter, the indications and outcomes of various modalities of radiation used to treat eyelid tumors (squamous cell carcinoma (SCC), basal cell carcinoma (BCC), sebaceous gland carcinoma, melanoma) and conjunctival tumors (SCC and melanoma) are discussed. Radiation therapy of ocular adnexal lymphoma is reviewed with orbital tumors [see chapter 'Radiation Therapy: Orbital Tumors' by Marwaha et al., this vol.].

Eyelid Tumors

Squamous Cell Carcinoma

Mohs micrographic surgery or wide excision with frozen section control is the primary treatment of choice for SCC of the eyelid [1, 2].

Indications

Advanced disease requiring substantial removal of tissue can result in poor cosmesis and loss of eyelid function. Radiation is an option for such patients and those who are unable to undergo extensive surgery due to other medical comorbidities.

Techniques and Results

• EBRT

In one series of 104 individuals with SCC of the eyelid treated with single or fractionated EBRT at doses of 20–60 Gy, the 5-year local tumor control rate was 93.3% [3].

• Brachytherapy

In some countries, an alternative approach for radiation therapy of SCC of the eyelid is the use of high dose rate interstitial brachytherapy. This technique uses a plastic tubing system inserted into the tumor to cover the target area. In one series of 10 patients with SCC of the eyelid treated with six fractions of 6.5 Gy over 6 days, a 90% 5-year disease-free survival was observed [4].

Basal Cell Carcinoma

While BCC of the eyelid can be locally invasive, it does not frequently metastasize. Surgical excision, Mohs micrographic surgery, and cryosurgery have been used to treat BCC with 5-year local control rates exceeding 90% [1, 2, 4].

Indications

The role of radiation therapy in the management of BCC is controversial, with some investigators reporting excellent control and others finding significant recurrence rates [5, 6]. For small and localized lesions, surgery is most frequently selected as primary therapy; however, radiation therapy is an attractive option for cases when surgical excision will result in severe loss of function or unacceptable cosmesis. This is particularly relevant to lesions affecting the inner canthus and lower eyelid where surgical treatment may result in scarring or damage to the lacrimal apparatus. When the decision is made to perform exenteration in cases with orbital invasion by periocular BCC, radiation can be used as adjuvant therapy [7].

Techniques and Results

• EBRT

One group has reported excellent results using EBRT in the treatment of a large series of 1062 BCC of the eyelid. Depending on tumor size, patients were treated with single or fractionated exposures to doses of 20–60 Gy. Using this scheme, the 5-year tumor control rate was 95% [3]. In the majority of these cases, a 5-day fractionated course of radiation to 35 Gy yielded excellent functional and cosmetic results. In the

5% of patients in whom recurrences developed, further radiation or surgery was effective in obtaining local tumor control [3]. Other investigators have cautioned against the use of radiation as primary therapy for periocular BCC. Recurrences, particularly those in the region of the midface are difficult to treat by any modality and carry a high risk of mortality [5].

• Brachytherapy
In some centers, high-dose-rate interstitial brachytherapy has been used for the treatment of BCC of the eyelid. In 2 patients treated with six fractions of 6.5 Gy over 6 days, a 50% 5-year disease-free survival was observed [4]. Other investigators have compared interstitial brachytherapy as well as other forms of radiation therapy to standard surgical excision for primary BCC of the face measuring less than 4 cm [6]. A study of 347 patients was conducted in which patients were either randomized to a surgery group or a radiation therapy group (55% were treated with interstitial brachytherapy, 33% with contact therapy, and 12% with conventional radiation therapy). The 4-year actuarial failure rate (95% CI) was 0.7% (0.1–3.9%) in the surgery group compared with 7.5% (4.2–13.1%) in the radiation therapy group. The cosmetic results were also assessed by independent observers and by the patients receiving treatment. In both cases, cosmesis was felt to be superior in those patients who underwent surgery. These findings suggest that radiation should be reserved as adjuvant therapy in appropriate cases [6].

Sebaceous Gland Carcinoma

Due to the aggressive clinical behavior of sebaceous gland carcinoma and potential for metastasis to regional lymph nodes and distant organs, the most acceptable primary therapy is complete surgical excision with wide margins.

Indications
Sebaceous gland carcinoma is not highly radiosensitive; however, in select advanced or diffuse cases, radiation may have a role as adjuvant or palliative therapy [8–10]. Radiation may be a potential treatment option; however, reports related to its use for sebaceous gland carcinoma are limited. Given the significant rate of treatment failure, short follow-up time for some patients, and the potential for delayed metastases, these studies again confirm that radiation is likely more appropriate as adjuvant therapy in sebaceous gland carcinoma [4, 11–13].

Techniques and Results
• EBRT
The role of EBRT as a curative therapy has been investigated by some groups (fig. 1) [11]. In one series of 10 patients with sebaceous gland carcinoma of the ocular adnexa,

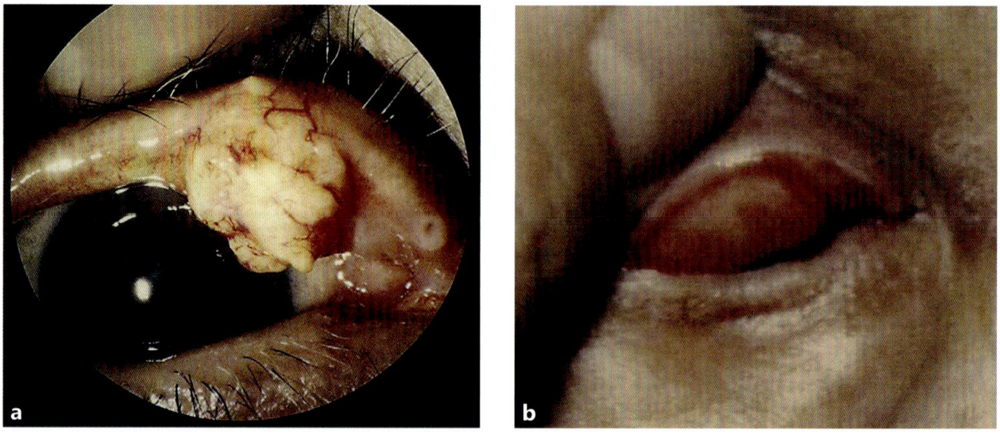

Fig. 1. Sebaceous gland carcinoma. Right upper eyelid before (**a**) and 2 weeks after irradiation (**b**). The yellowish and cauliflower-like tumor (arrowheads) has completely disappeared. The radiation protocol included total doses of 50–66.6 Gy (median, 60 Gy) delivered in 22–37 fractions (median, 29 fractions), with fraction sizes of 1.8 to 2.2 Gy (median, 2 Gy) for 5 days per week. Reproduced with permission from Hata et al. [12].

four patients were treated definitively at a dose of 45–63 Gy over 4–7 weeks. The remaining 6 patients received postoperative radiation therapy to the parotid bed and ipsilateral cervical lymph node chain for parotid metastases, which developed within 36 months of initial surgical treatment. Local control was 90% after a follow-up ranging from 2 to 10 years, and overall disease specific actuarial survival was 96% at 5 years [11].

• Brachytherapy
High-dose-rate interstitial brachytherapy has also been explored in some centers as a potential treatment of sebaceous gland carcinoma of the eyelid [4]. In one series of 8 cases of sebaceous gland carcinoma treated with six fractions of 6.5 Gy over 6 days, a 5-year disease-free survival of 57% was observed [4].

Eyelid Melanoma

For small, circumscribed malignant melanoma of the eyelid, surgical excision with wide margins is the recommended therapy [14]. This is generally followed by plastics repair and exenteration for large or diffuse neoplasms [15].

Indications
Radiation therapy has been used following surgery in cases where residual disease is present at the margins of resection [16]. It has also been used as an alternative to exenteration in select cases [14].

Techniques and Results

• EBRT

EBRT has been used in some centers when regional lymph node metastases are detected following wide local excision; however, the small number of patients treated precludes meaningful analysis of outcomes [17].

• Brachytherapy

In one series, 14 patients, all of whom had undergone previous debulking, incomplete resection, or recurrence following surgery, were treated with ^{125}I brachytherapy. A stainless steel pericorneal ring eye shield was used in combination with ^{125}I seeds in polythene tubes inserted into the eyelid. A median dose of 37 Gy (range 17.3–67.6 Gy) was delivered over the course of 113 h (range 47–190 h) to the outer surface of target tumor volume [14]. Local control was achieved in thirteen patients after a median follow-up of 39 months. There were two recurrences at 8 and 13 months in 1 patient who received 17.3 Gy. Three patients subsequently died with metastatic disease at 44, 62 and 79 months following brachytherapy [14].

Conjunctival Tumors

Squamous Cell Carcinoma

Surgical excision is traditionally the most frequently employed primary treatment for SCC of the conjunctiva [18]. Adjuvant treatment with cryotherapy is commonly used in conjunction with surgery, and chemotherapy may be used for selected cases such as those with residual conjunctival disease.

Indications

Radiation therapy may be indicated in some circumstances, for example when pathology demonstrates scleral invasion of conjunctival SCC following excision, or in cases of persistently recurrent disease. It may also be used in cases of advanced SCC with intraocular extension, orbital extension, or when surgery is not a curative option. Radiation therapy is generally deferred until after the conjunctiva or primary surgical site has healed. Various radiation modalities and treatment regimens have been employed for conjunctival SCC.

Techniques and Results

• EBRT

EBRT utilizing photons, electrons, and protons alone, or in combination has been used for both curative and palliative treatment for unresponsive and progressive SCC [3, 19–22]. In one series of 8 patients with conjunctival SCC who had failed multiple standard treatments and underwent EBRT (dosed in a range of 50–60 Gy

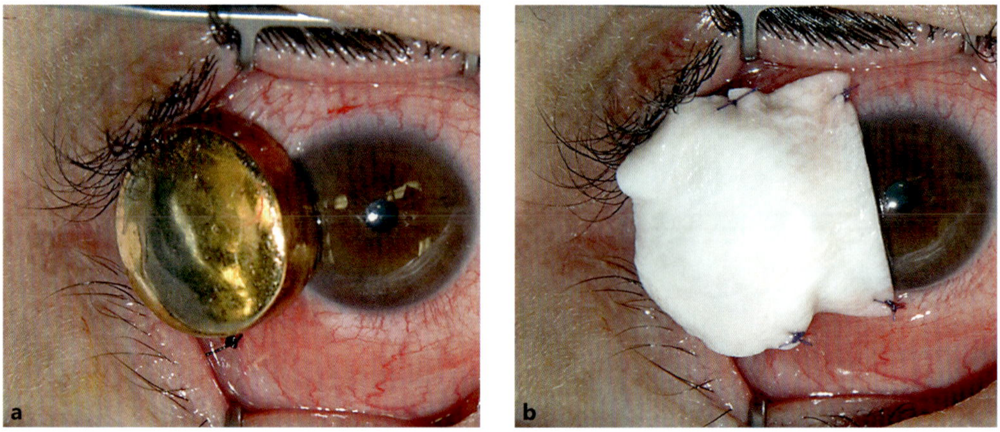

Fig. 2. Invasive conjunctival squamous cell carcinoma with extension into sclera treated with ^{125}I brachytherapy (45 Gy to the depth of 3 mm) (**a**). The plaque was covered with donor pericardium (**b**) followed by temporary transmarginal tarsorrhaphy to minimize postoperative discomfort for the duration of the implant placement (48 h). Reproduced with permission from Pe'er and Frucht-Pery [35].

in 2.0- to 2.5-Gy daily fractions), local tumor control and regression were noted in 6 patients (75%) and recurrences were noted in 2. No metastatic spread or tumor-related deaths occurred after a median follow-up of 30.25 months [23].

For lesions involving the palpebral conjunctiva and fornix, higher radiation doses may be required to achieve local control. For such patients, proton therapy is an option and can be given at a dose of 32 Gy in six fractions followed by a boost to the tumor bed of 14 Gy in 2 fractions [24]. Rarely, intraocular invasion from conjunctival SCC can occur. There are reports of such cases being successfully treated using proton beam therapy employing a total dose of 32 Gy, in 8 Gy divided fractions on 4 consecutive days [25].

• Brachytherapy

Brachytherapy, most commonly with ^{90}Sr, has been used at a dose of 20–180 Gy to the tumor surface [26]. Radiation administration with a hand-held ^{90}Sr applicator delivering 60 Gy to the tumor surface in four fractions once a week, or 50 Gy in five daily fractions has also resulted in excellent tumor control [24]. For tumors larger than an available hand-held applicator, or those with scleral invasion, ^{125}I radioactive plaque can be employed (fig. 2) [24]. One recommended dose for ^{125}I plaque is 60 Gy at a depth of 2–3 mm [24]. Other investigators have used a treatment dose was 100 Gy to a depth of 1.5–2.5 mm to treat conjunctival SCC following excision for cases with evidence of scleral invasion [27]. After 23.4 months of follow up, no patients experienced recurrence at the primary treatment site, however one individual developed a new lesion distant from the initial site of therapy [27]. In treatment centers where ^{106}Ru is available, the plaque can be applied immediately following excision to deliver a dose of 130 Gy at a depth of 2 mm, or after the conjunctiva has healed using a dose of 100 Gy at a depth of 1–2 mm [24, 28]. Another treatment algorithm for ^{106}Ru is a dose of 320 Gy delivered to the tumor bed. Using this treatment scheme, local control has been achieved (follow-up of 22 months) without major complications from radiation. Recurrence rates following brachytherapy have ranged from 2 to 47%, therefore brachytherapy alone is typically not recommended as primary therapy [18].

Conjunctival Melanoma

Primary treatment for conjunctival melanoma typically involves complete excision with surgical margins of 3–5 mm when possible [29]. Adjuvant treatments using cryotherapy to the surgical margins and/or tumor bed as well as absolute alcohol epitheliectomy for corneal and limbal involvement are frequently combined with surgery.

Indications

Radiation therapy may also be used as an adjuvant treatment following primary resection. In general, conjunctival melanoma is not radiosensitive, and therefore radiation should not be used as a sole therapy [30]. Radiation therapy may also be indicated for certain circumstances including deep scleral invasion detected by pathology following primary excision, recurrent disease unresponsive to other therapies, palliation for extensive disease which is not surgically excisable, or in patients who cannot tolerate surgery.

Techniques and Results

- EBRT

EBRT has been used as adjuvant radiation therapy (total dose of 60 Gy) in tumors with high risk features such as increased thickness or close margins of resection [19, 31].

Proton beam radiation has also been investigated as an alternative to exenteration for diffuse and multifocal patterns of conjunctival melanoma which are not treatable with standard eye-sparing methods [32]. In one series of 20 patients, areas of the conjunctiva with suspected microscopic disease were treated by 31 Gy in 6 fractions. High-risk regions of the conjunctiva with clinically detectable tumor were treated by an additional boost using a smaller beam size and applying 2 fractions up to 45 Gy. An individually shaped compensator was brought into the beam to modify the range of the protons so that the eye was irradiated at a depth of 2 mm. After a median follow-up of 34 months, recurrent disease occurred in 6 cases (30%); 2 of these were outside the irradiated volume, 3 were within the target volume treated by 31 Gy, and 1 was in the primary target volume treated by 45 Gy. Exenteration was eventually necessary in

2 patients (10%). Six patients (30%) developed metastatic disease and 4 (20%) deaths occurred suggesting that proton beam therapy should be used with caution in advanced cases of conjunctival melanoma [32, 33].

• Brachytherapy

When brachytherapy is used as adjuvant treatment following excision, one group has advocated for using either ^{90}Sr or ^{90}Y with a 10-Gy daily dose applied at the tumor surface until a total dose of 150–200 Gy is delivered, depending on the thickness of the neoplasm [30]. In one series of 19 patients treated with ^{125}I plaque (treatment dose of 100 Gy to a depth of 1.5–3.0 mm) following surgical resection, there were no recurrences at the initial treatment site or metastases after a median follow-up of 43.1 months; however, 3 individuals developed new lesions at a site distant from the primary location [34].

For malignant melanoma affecting the palpebral conjunctiva and fornix, ^{125}I plaque application following tumor excision has been successfully employed using a dosing schedule of 100 Gy in 4 weekly fractions of 25 Gy [24]. An alternative approach is brachytherapy using ^{125}I seeds within the eyelid. A perilimbal stainless steel shield attached to the extraocular muscles can be used to protect the cornea and lens. Using this method and a dose of 55–60 Gy delivered over 5 days, one group showed excellent local control in 13 of 14 patients [14].

Conclusions

It is important to note that the majority of experience using radiation to treat eyelid and conjunctival tumors is based upon results from small case series. It is therefore difficult to assess overall efficacy and optimal treatment protocols for incorporating radiation into the treatment planning of these tumors. Furthermore, the rare nature of these tumors, varying tumor classification schemes, and confounding prognostic clinical factors such as tumor size and location contribute to the difficulty in analyzing outcomes following radiation.

References

1 Mohs FE: Micrographic surgery for the microscopically controlled excision of eyelid cancers. Arch Ophthalmol 1986;104:901–909.

2 Malhotra R, Huilgol SC, Huynh NT, Selva D: The Australian Mohs database: periocular squamous cell carcinoma. Ophthalmology 2004;111:617–623.

3 Fitzpatrick PJ, Thompson GA, Easterbrook WM, et al: Basal and squamous cell carcinoma of the eyelids and their treatment by radiotherapy. Int J Radiat Oncol Biol Phys 1984;10:449–454.

4 Azad S, Choudhary V: Treatment results of high dose rate interstitial brachytherapy in carcinoma of eye lid. J Cancer Res Ther 2011;7:157–161.

5 Margo CE, Waltz K: Basal cell carcinoma of the eyelid and periocular skin. Surv Ophthalmol 1993;38: 169–192.

6 Avril MF, Auperin A, Margulis A, et al: Basal cell carcinoma of the face: surgery or radiotherapy? Results of a randomized study. Br J Cancer 1997;76: 100–106.

7 Leibovitch I, McNab A, Sullivan T, et al: Orbital invasion by periocular basal cell carcinoma. Ophthalmology 2005;112:717–723.
8 Shields JA, Demirci H, Marr BP, et al: Sebaceous carcinoma of the ocular region: a review. Surv Ophthalmol 2005;50:103–122.
9 Yen MT, Tse DT, Wu X, Wolfson AH: Radiation therapy for local control of eyelid sebaceous cell carcinoma: report of two cases and review of the literature. Ophthal Plast Reconstr Surg 2000;16:211–215.
10 Murthy R, Honavar SG, Burman S, et al: Neoadjuvant chemotherapy in the management of sebaceous gland carcinoma of the eyelid with regional lymph node metastasis. Ophthal Plast Reconstr Surg 2005;21:307–309.
11 Pardo FS, Borodic G: Long-term follow-up of patients undergoing definitive radiation therapy for sebaceous carcinoma of the ocular adnexae. Int J Radiat Oncol Biol Phys 1996;34:1189–1190.
12 Hata M, Koike I, Omura M, et al: Noninvasive and curative radiation therapy for sebaceous carcinoma of the eyelid. Int J Radiat Oncol Biol Phys 2012;82: 605–611.
13 Hendley RL, Rieser JC, Cavanagh HD, et al: Primary radiation therapy for meibomian gland carcinoma. Am J Ophthalmol 1979;87:206–209.
14 Stannard CE, Sealy GR, Hering ER, et al: Malignant melanoma of the eyelid and palpebral conjunctiva treated with iodine-125 brachytherapy. Ophthalmology 2000;107:951–958.
15 Hungerford JL: Management of ocular melanoma. Br Med Bull 1995;51:694–716.
16 Lederman M: Radiotherapy of malignant melanomata of the eye. Br J Radiol 1961;34:21–42.
17 Esmaeli B, Wang B, Deavers M, et al: Prognostic factors for survival in malignant melanoma of the eyelid skin. Ophthal Plast Reconstr Surg 2000;16:250–257.
18 Pe'er J, Frucht-Pery J: Ocular surface squamous neoplasia; in Singh AD, Damato BE, Pe'er J, Murphree AL, Perry JD (eds): Clinical Ophthalmic Oncology. Philadelphia, Saunders-Elsevier, 2007.
19 Hsu A, Frank SJ, Ballo MT, et al: Postoperative adjuvant external-beam radiation therapy for cancers of the eyelid and conjunctiva. Ophthal Plast Reconstr Surg 2008;24:444–449.
20 Caujolle JP, Maschi C, Chauvel P, et al: Surgery and additional protontherapy for treatment of invasive and recurrent squamous cell carcinomas: technique and preliminary results. J Fr Ophtalmol 2009;32:707–714.
21 Sinesi C, McNeese MD, Peters LJ, et al: Electron beam therapy for eyelid carcinomas. Head Neck Surg 1987;10:31–37.
22 Bowyer JD, Sullivan TJ, Whitehead KJ, et al: The management of perineural spread of squamous cell carcinoma to the ocular adnexae. Ophthal Plast Reconstr Surg 2003;19:275–281.
23 Graue GF, Tena LB, Finger PT: Electron beam radiation for conjunctival squamous carcinoma. Ophthal Plast Reconstr Surg 2011;27:277–281.
24 Stannard C, Sauerwein W, Maree G, Lecuona K: Radiotherapy for ocular tumours. Eye (Lond) 2013;27: 119–127.
25 Ramonas KM, Conway RM, Daftari IK, et al: Successful treatment of intraocularly invasive conjunctival squamous cell carcinoma with proton beam therapy. Arch Ophthalmol 2006;124:126–128.
26 Lommatzsch P: Beta-ray treatment of malignant epithelial tumors of the conjunctiva. Am J Ophthalmol 1976;81:198–206.
27 Walsh-Conway N, Conway RM: Plaque brachytherapy for the management of ocular surface malignancies with corneoscleral invasion. Clin Exp Ophthalmol 2009;37:577–583.
28 Damato B, Coupland SE: An audit of conjunctival melanoma treatment in Liverpool. Eye (Lond) 2009; 23:801–809.
29 Pe'er J, Frucht-Pery J: Conjunctival melanoma; in Singh AD, Damato BE, Pe'er J, Murphree AL, Perry JD (eds): Clinical Ophthalmic Oncology. Philadelphia, Saunders-Elsevier, 2007.
30 Lommatzsch PK, Lommatzsch RE, Kirsch I, Fuhrmann P: Therapeutic outcome of patients suffering from malignant melanomas of the conjunctiva. Br J Ophthalmol 1990;74:615–619.
31 Savar A, Esmaeli B, Ho H, et al: Conjunctival melanoma: local-regional control rates, and impact of high-risk histopathologic features. J Cutan Pathol 2011;38:18–24.
32 Wuestemeyer H, Sauerwein W, Meller D, et al: Proton radiotherapy as an alternative to exenteration in the management of extended conjunctival melanoma. Graefes Arch Clin Exp Ophthalmol 2006;244: 438–446.
33 Henkind P: Conjunctival melanocytic lesions: natural history; in Jakobiec FA (ed): Ocular and Adnexal Tumors. Birmingham, Aesculapius, 1978.
34 Karim R, Conway RM: Conservative resection and adjuvant plaque brachytherapy for early-stage conjunctival melanoma. Clin Exp Ophthalmol 2011;39: 293–298.
35 Pe'er J, Frucht-Pery J: Squamous Neoplasia. Clinical Ophthalmic Oncology, ed 2. Conjunctival and Corneal Tumors. Berlin, Springer, 2013.

Arun D. Singh, MD
Director, Department of Ophthalmic Oncology, Cole Eye Institute
Cleveland Clinic Foundation, 9500 Euclid Avenue
Cleveland, OH 44195 (USA)
E-Mail singha@ccf.org

Singh AD, Pelayes DE, Seregard S, Macklis R (eds): Ophthalmic Radiation Therapy. Techniques and Applications.
Dev Ophthalmol. Basel, Karger, 2013, vol 52, pp 94–101 (DOI: 10.1159/000351084)

Radiation Therapy: Orbital Tumors

Gaurav Marwaha[a] · Roger Macklis[a] · Arun D. Singh[b]

[a]Department of Radiation Oncology, Taussig Cancer Center and [b]Department of Ophthalmic Oncology, Cole Eye Institute, Cleveland Clinic Foundation, Cleveland, Ohio, USA

Abstract

Orbital tumors are rare overall, comprising 0.1% of all tumors and less than 20% of all orbital diseases. Tumors may be benign, locally aggressive, or malignant. Of the malignant tumors, lymphomas and metastases are the most common and are primarily seen in the elderly population. While surgery and chemotherapeutic agents are often employed in the management of these lesions, not all patients are candidates for these therapies. Radiation therapy offers a noninvasive, well-tolerated primary treatment modality, whereby vision-sparing is feasible in many cases. In this chapter, we review an array of non-neoplastic entities and orbital tumors, for which there exists a role for radiation, and the radiotherapeutic techniques and applications in their management.

Orbital tumors are rare overall, comprising 0.1% of all tumors and less than 20% of all orbital diseases [1]. The orbit is the bony protective cone-shaped cavity in which ocular functional structures are contained. It is comprised of seven bones, with an average volume in adults of 30 ml, and medial length × width × height of 45 × 40 × 35 mm [2]. Within the orbit, the following structures are found: the globe, extraocular muscles, fat, vessels, nerve, glands, and connective tissue.

Tumors may arise from any of these structures, and they may be primary, secondary (through invasion from another structure), or metastatic in nature. Primary tumors, specifically, may be myogenic, melanocytic, lipomatous/myxomatous, fibroblastic, histiocytic, or can arise from the vasculature, lacrimal gland, bone, lymphocytes, or peripheral nerve/sheath. Secondary orbital tumors occur when the orbit is invaded by tumors arising from sites like the eyelids, lacrimal sac, conjuctiva, paranasal sinuses, globe, brain, or nasopharynx [2]. Metastases may be from any primary site in the body, most frequently cancers of the breast, lung, unknown primary, and prostate.

Patients may present with various clinical findings, including the more common exophthalmos and/or proptosis, but also with visual problems (double vision or visual loss), pain, or pressure. Radiotherapy is an effective means by which to treat orbital tumors for cure or palliation, while preserving function of vision critical structures, and ultimately quality of life. The treatment paradigm for benign disease is usually surgical resection, with radiation reserved for salvage. On the other hand, the pendulum has swung, for the most part, in favor of primary radiotherapy in the treatment of malignant orbital tumors.

Non-Neoplastic Entities

Graves' Ophthalmopathy

In approximately 1/3 of patients with the autoimmune Graves' disease, inflammation of the orbital tissues, known as Graves' ophthalmopathy, can occur. Over time, this can manifest as exophthalmos, ophthalmoplegia, extraocular muscle dysfunction, diplopia, blurred vision, eyelid and periorbital edema, lid lag and retraction, and compressive optic neuropathy. Graves' ophthalmopathy is believed to be an autoimmune disease in which activated T lymphocytes invade the orbit and stimulate glycosaminoglycan production in fibroblasts, which results in tissue edema, lymphocytic infiltration, and marked enlargement of the extraocular muscles.

First-line treatment includes high-dose steroids for at least 2 weeks, or surgical orbital decompression. Surgery is especially preferred when there is rapidly progressive optic neuropathy or severe proptosis. Radiation therapy can be employed for persistent disease or for patients in which steroids are contraindicated. Optimal radiation prescription is a dosage of 20 Gy/10 fx, prescribed with 4–6 MV photons via opposed lateral beams and half-beam blocks [3]. Some advocate for smaller doses per fraction; 20 Gy at 1 Gy/fx given over 20 weeks, for example, was shown to be more effective and better tolerated than 20 Gy at 2 Gy/fx in a German study [4]. Fields should encompass the muscles up to the insertion at the orbital apex and with an anterior edge just posterior to the lens. Concurrent steroids are generally given, and have been shown to be beneficial in symptomatic relief versus radiation alone in various randomized trials [5]. Seventy to 75% of patients receiving 20 Gy respond positively or require no further steroid therapy, and roughly 50% of patients have improvement in proptosis [5].

Orbital Pseudotumor

Orbital pseudotumor is an idiopathic inflammatory condition of the orbit (unilateral or bilateral) that may or may not involve the lacrimal gland. Extensive inflammatory infiltration produces acute pain, injected conjunctiva, periorbital swelling, decreased ocular motility, and exophathalmos. Histopathologically, there is mixed cellular infiltrate made up of lymphocytes, plasma cells, eosinophils, and polymorphonuclear leukocytes. While the pseudotumor can resolve on its own, nonsurgical treatments are often employed in order to prevent visual loss. Steroids are usually initiated first and foremost, with half of patients exhibiting some response within a few days [5]. Radiation therapy enhances local control rates to >75%. Anterior, lateral, or oblique treatment fields (^{60}Co, 4–6 MV photons, or 15–16 MeV electrons) are used for treatment, with a standard fractionation prescription dose of 20–25 Gy. As the lens is at very high risk for radiation damage, at institutions like MD Anderson, lens blocking is performed with a lead contact lens to minimize lens dose to well under its 7-Gy tolerance [5].

Benign Tumors

Optic Pathway Glioma

These tumors are considered as low-grade astroyctic tumors, comprising 5% of childhood brain tumors [6]. Greater than 75% occur in children under the age of 10 years. Thirty percent of optic pathway glioma patients have NF1 and up to 25% of NF1 patients develop optic pathway glioma, making it the most common CNS tumor in NF1. Anterior or prechiasmal lesions are more common in very young children, and posterior lesions (anterior 3rd ventricle, hypothalamus, and chiasm) occur more commonly in adolescents and tend to have a worse prognosis.

Children are generally managed with observation and close follow-up if feasible, whereas adults are managed more aggressively. First-line treatment for children is carboplatin/vincrisitine combination chemotherapy, reserving radiation for failure, whereas adults are primarily treated with radiation (fig. 1) [7]. Radiation doses range from 45 to 56 Gy, in 1.8 Gy/fx. For children under 3 years of age, a dose of 45 Gy is adequate, though chemotherapy is preferred if patients are <7 years old. This is because the risk for secondary malignancy is much greater in younger patients, and particularly high in patients with NF1 [8]. Doses ranging from 50 to 56 Gy are fitting for patients above the age of ten (fig. 2).

Meningioma

Meningiomas represent the second most common primary intracranial tumors [9]. Incidence increases with age, with the mean age being 56 years. Risk factors include exposure to ionizing radiation and also being female, which is associated with 2–3 times the relative risk. Forty percent of sporadic meningiomas occur in patients with neurofibromatosis 2. The majority, 78%, are benign, or WHO grade I. WHO

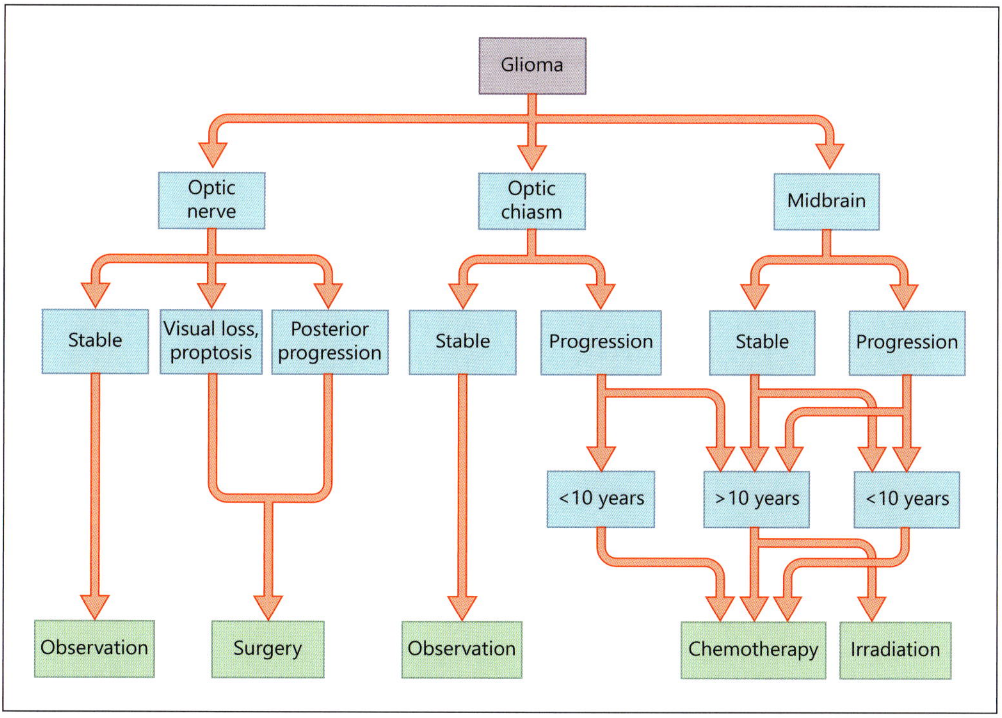

Fig. 1. Optic pathway gliomas. Reproduced with permission from Dutton [6].

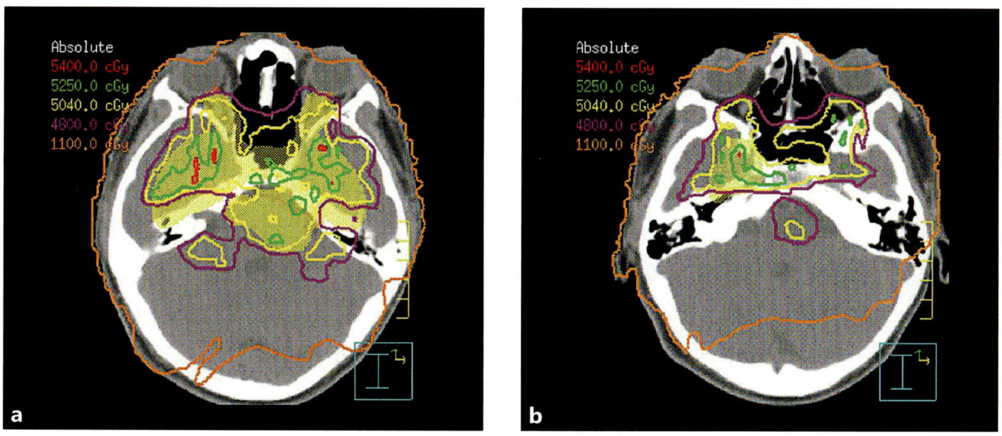

Fig. 2. Optic pathway gliomas. 12-year-old male with NF-1 and bilateral optic gliomas s/p multiple chemotherapy regimens, who developed progressive disease, now being treated with radiation therapy: 5,040 cGy in 28 fx to bilateral optic pathways. Superior (**a**) and just inferior (**b**) transverse slices of the intensity modulated radiation treatment plan. Note that the conformal dose distribution covering the target volume (yellow line) is confined to the affected tissues.

grades II and III comprise 20% and <2% of tumors, respectively [10]. Primary orbital meningiomas account for 1.3% of all meningiomas [11]. When they occur primarily within the orbit, they tend to arise from optic nerve sheath or the sphenoid bone [11].

Optic nerve sheath meningiomas most often present with progressive unilateral visual loss, proptosis, and limited ocular motility. These are very slow-growing tumors that grow within the subarachnoid space, eventually encapsulating the nerve itself. The mean age for presentation is 41 years, and the prognosis is generally very good given their often indolent nature [11]. On T1-weighted gadolinium enhanced MRI, these meningiomas appear isointense or hypointense to gray matter, and on T2-weighted gadolinium enhanced MRI, they appear isointense or hyperintense. The optic nerve and sheath are thickened when compared to orbital fat, with increased signal intensity compared with normal optic nerve [6].

The mainstay of treatment for meningiomas, including those arising from the sphenoid wing, is surgical resection [6]. Note that observation can be considered for meningiomas confined to the intraorbital optic nerve, in the setting of stable clinical and radiographic findings. Radiation therapy, when indicated, is the preferred primary treatment modality in vision preservation. The patient should be simulated supine with IV contrast, thermoplastic mask, and isocenter placed in the middle of the tumor [see chapter 'Teletherapy: Advanced Techniques' by Stockham et al., this vol.]. At the Cleveland Clinic, standard fractionation is with 50.4 Gy/28 fractions at 1.8 Gy/fx, using IMRT, generally with 6-MV photons and with 5–7 mm margins on GTV. This is a slightly lower dose than the 54 Gy often used for other, more common intracranial sites, in an effort to preserve useful vision. SRS should not be utilized for treatment of optic nerve sheath meningiomas as there is considerable risk for blindness with this modality.

Malignant Tumors

Orbital and Adnexal Lymphoma

Non-Hodgkin lymphoma of the orbit is very rare, comprising roughly 1% of all non-Hodgkin lymphoma cases and 10% of all tumors of the orbit [5]. These tumors arise from the conjunctiva of the eye, and are generally asymptomatic. Histology is generally MALT (mucosa-associated lymphoid tissue) or follicular B cell lymphoma, and they usually present as localized, stage IE. Vision is generally not affected, but these tumors can cause exophthalmos, pain, diplopia, and swelling. Standard work-up should include CT or MRI of the orbit as well as bone marrow biopsies and CT chest/abdomen/pelvis for complete staging.

Treatment for localized, low-grade lymphomas consists of external beam radiotherapy (fig. 3). Treatment for high-grade diffuse large B cell lymphoma involves

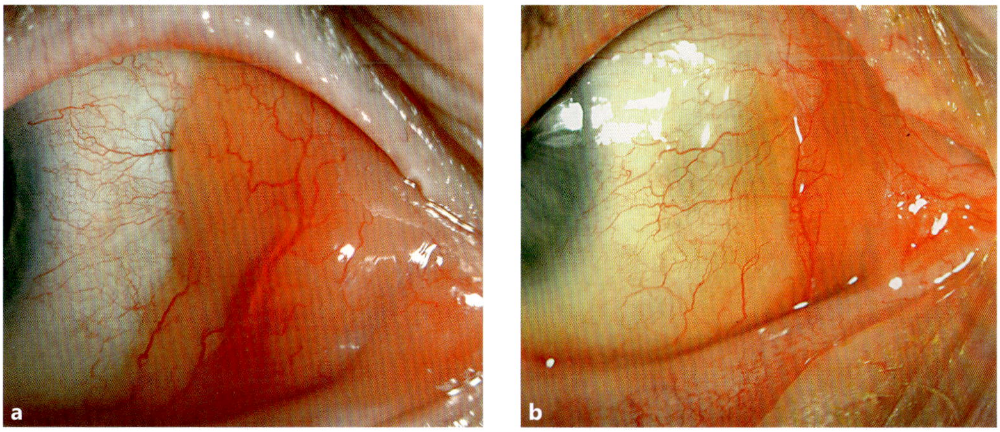

Fig. 3. Concomitant involvement of the conjunctiva by MALT lymphoma and small lymphocytic lymphoma associated with IgM macroglobulinemia. **a** Right eye lesion pre-IMRT. **b** Right eye lesion post-IMRT.

induction chemotherapy, usually with R-CHOP, followed by consolidative radiotherapy. For radiation planning, the patient is set up supine, with a thermoplastic mask for head immobilization. Doses for MALT are 25–32.4 Gy in 1.8 Gy/fx [5]. For low-grade lymphoma (MALT lymphoma), 30 Gy is ideal. For consolidation of high-grade lymphomas status postchemotherapy, response-adapted radiation therapy is ideal, whereby 30 Gy is reasonable for complete responders and 36–40 Gy is recommended for partial responders. Electron beam treatment using 6–9 MeV and 0.5–1.0 cm bolus is recommended for anterior lesions. Photons are generally required for deeper, posterior lesions. The cornea and lens may be in particular risk for radiation toxicity, but institutions differ in their usage of shielding. The Cleveland Clinic does not utilize shielding, for example, whereas MD Anderson Cancer Center, shields with 3 mm of tungsten in order to reduce corneal and lens doses to <5% [5]. IMRT is another way to decrease toxicity (fig. 4). Response to radiation therapy tends to be excellent. In a study by Fung CY et al. [12], 5-year local control rates were >80% with doses under 30 Gy and was 100% with higher doses. Long-term follow-up is paramount in these patients, as extraorbital metastases can be seen in even the lowest grade, MALT lymphomas, at rates of nearly 20–50% at 5 years [13].

Lacrimal Gland Tumors

These tumors comprise <15% of all orbital tumors, with benign tumors usually comprised of pleomorphic adenoma and malignant as adenoid cystic carcinoma or malignant mixed tumors. Most occur in middle-age with equal sex incidence.

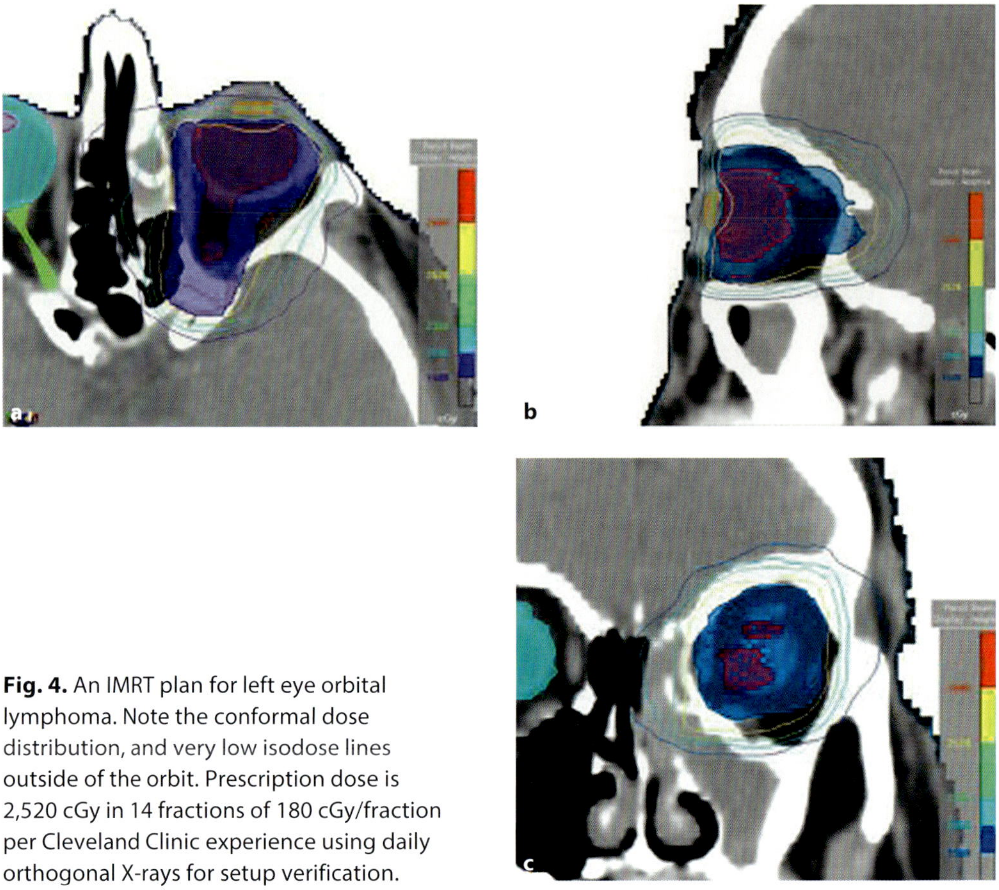

Fig. 4. An IMRT plan for left eye orbital lymphoma. Note the conformal dose distribution, and very low isodose lines outside of the orbit. Prescription dose is 2,520 cGy in 14 fractions of 180 cGy/fraction per Cleveland Clinic experience using daily orthogonal X-rays for setup verification.

They tend to present with eyelid swelling or a mass, where malignant tumors tend to have a shorter history and more painful course [14]. Pleomorphic adenomas are addressed with surgery alone, but adenoid cystic carcinomas and malignant mixed tumors are treated with debulking surgery followed by external beam radiation therapy. Doses of 55–60 Gy are adequate for adenoid cystic carcinomas after surgical debulking, with median disease-free survival of 3 years and median survival of 10 years [15]. Similar dosing should be used for malignant mixed tumors. Radiation fields should include the following parts of the orbit: lacrimal fossa, orbital apex, superior orbital fissure, anterior cavernous sinus, and superolateral soft tissues [14].

References

1 Taban M, Perry JD: Classification of orbital tumors; in Singh AD, Damato BE, Pe'er J, et al (eds): Clinical Ophthalmic Oncology. Phildelphia, Saunders-Elsevier, 2007.

2 Mercandetti M: Orbital tumors. Medscape reference: drugs, diseases and procedures. 2011. Available online: http://emedicine.medscape.com/article/1218892-overview.

3 Prummel MF, Terwee CB, Gerding MN, et al: A randomized controlled trial of orbital radiotherapy versus sham irradiation in patients with mild Graves' ophthalmopathy. J Clin Endocrinol Metab 2004;89: 15–20.

4 Kahaly GJ, Rosler HP, Pitz S, Hommel G: Low- versus high-dose radiotherapy for Graves' ophthalmopathy: a randomized, single blind trial. J Clin Endocrinol Metab 2000;85:102–108.

5 Schwartz DL, Kim SK, Ang KK: The orbit; in Cox JD, Ang KKE (eds): Radiation Oncology: Rationale, Technique, Results, ed 9. Philadelphia, Mosby Elsevier, 2010.

6 Dutton JJ: Tumors of the optic nerve; in Singh AD, Damato BE, Pe'er J, et al (eds): Clinical Ophthalmic Oncology. Phildelphia, Saunders-Elsevier, 2007.

7 Jahraus CD, Tarbell NJ: Optic pathway gliomas. Pediatr Blood Cancer 2006;46:586–596.

8 Sharif S, Ferner R, Birch JM, et al: Second primary tumors in neurofibromatosis 1 patients treated for optic glioma: substantial risks after radiotherapy. J Clin Oncol 2006;24:2570–2575.

9 Claus EB, Bondy ML, Schildkraut JM, et al: Epidemiology of intracranial meningioma. Neurosurgery 2005; 57:1088–1095.

10 Willis J, Smith C, Ironside JW, et al: The accuracy of meningioma grading: a 10-year retrospective audit. Neuropathol Appl Neurobiol 2005;31:141–149.

11 Patel BCK: Benign tumors of the orbit; in Singh AD, Damato BE, Pe'er J, et al (eds): Clinical Ophthalmic Oncology. Phildelphia, Saunders-Elsevier, 2007.

12 Fung CY, Tarbell NJ, Lucarelli MJ, et al: Ocular adnexal lymphoma: clinical behavior of distinct World Health Organization classification subtypes. Int J Radiat Oncol Biol, Phys 2003;57:1382–1391.

13 Jenkins C, Rose GE, Bunce C, et al: Histological features of ocular adnexal lymphoma (REAL classification) and their association with patient morbidity and survival. Br J Ophthalmol 2000;84:907–913.

14 Durrani OM, Rose GE: Tumors of the lacrimal gland; in Singh AD, Damato BE, Pe'er J, et al (eds): Clinical Ophthalmic Oncology. Phildelphia, Saunders-Elsevier, 2007.

15 Esmaeli B, Ahmadi MA, Youssef A, et al: Outcomes in patients with adenoid cystic carcinoma of the lacrimal gland. Ophthal Plastic Reconstr Surg 2004;20: 22–26.

Gaurav Marwaha, MD
Department of Radiation Oncology, Cleveland Clinic Foundation
9500 Euclid Avenue T-28
Cleveland, OH 44195 (USA)
E-Mail marwahg2@ccf.org

Singh AD, Pelayes DE, Seregard S, Macklis R (eds): Ophthalmic Radiation Therapy. Techniques and Applications. Dev Ophthalmol. Basel, Karger, 2013, vol 52, pp 102–113 (DOI: 10.1159/000351087)

Radiation Therapy: Anterior Segment Complications

Carlos A. Medina Mendez[a] · Arun D. Singh[b]

[a]Vitreoretinal Service, and [b]Department of Ophthalmic Oncology, Cole Eye Institute, Cleveland Clinic Foundation, Cleveland, Ohio, USA

Abstract

The goal of radiotherapy is to produce maximal damage to the tumor yet at the same time produce minimal damage to the surrounding tissues. Here we discuss anterior chamber complications of radiotherapy. These can vary from ocular surface irritation to blindness and can be subdivided into acute (<4 weeks) and chronic (>4 weeks). Prevention and management is also discussed and subdivided by affected tissue.

The goal of radiotherapy is to produce maximal damage to the tumor yet at the same time produce minimal damage to the surrounding tissues [1]. Radiotherapy complications can vary from ocular surface irritation to blindness [2, 3]. The development of complications varies depending on a number of factors. Tissue tolerance to radiation is an important factor for consideration in the planning and execution of treatment [4].

In general, acute radiation effects (<4 weeks) mostly develop involving the anterior segment while chronic or late (>4 weeks) effects are confined to the posterior segment and orbital tissues [4]. Acute lesions are primarily due to radiation effects on rapidly proliferating cells such as those present in the eyelid skin, conjunctiva and corneal epithelium [2]. It has also been hypothesized that radiation is more harmful in children because of the rapid growth of normal tissue [1, 2]. With proper medical management, recovery from mild forms of radiation injury generally occurs within several weeks after the completion of the treatment.

Delayed complications may follow acute injury and may present years after radiotherapy. The pathogenic mechanisms include endothelial cell damage including damage to the retinal microcirculation with passage of proteinaceous fluid into the interstitial spaces as well as edema and subsequent fibrosis of the tissue [5]. In this chapter, we review the acute and late complications of radiation to the ocular adnexa, ocular surface and anterior chamber. Posterior segment complications are discussed elsewhere [chapter by Seregard et al., this vol.].

Eyelids and Periocular Skin

Acute

As the eyelid skin is the thinnest in the body, it is not uncommon for patients to complain of redness, surface peeling, burning, itching and pain. Erythema lasting for a few days can occur within hours of treatment and is more commonly seen in males, increasing age and sun-exposed skin (fig. 1). Desquamation and scaling can occur after 1 week of therapy with doses of more than or equal to 10 Gy [1]. Blisters and edema may be followed by moist dermatitis [6]. This is uncommon in doses of less than 40 Gy and presents with exposure of the dermis and serum leakage. Desquamation may lead to secondary infection and long-term scarring [3]. Epilation is commonly reversible and is usually present very early after treatment but may also appear in later stages and be permanent (fig. 2). It usually occurs with cumulative doses of >20 Gy but can occur with doses as low as 10 Gy delivered over 3 days [7].

Late

Late radiation effects to the eyelids and periorbital skin include epilation, telangiectasia, pigmentary changes, hyperkeratosis, atrophy, necrosis, ulceration, punctual occlusion, cicatricial ectropion, ptosis and other eyelid deformities [1]. Late effects like hyperpigmentation and telangiectasia usually occur more than 1 year after treatment [8].

Management

Effects of radiation to the eyelids and periorbital areas should be treated aggressively. Topical antibiotics should be used in the presence of any open wounds. Topical corticosteroids (1% hydrocortisone) may be beneficial but should be used cautiously because of side effects that include cataracts and glaucoma. If periocular steroids are used intraocular pressure must be monitored regularly. In severe cases, wound debridement and rarely reconstructive surgery may be needed.

In all cases, the patient should be instructed to wash the eyelids with mild soap and warm water. Care should be taken while drying to prevent any significant trau-

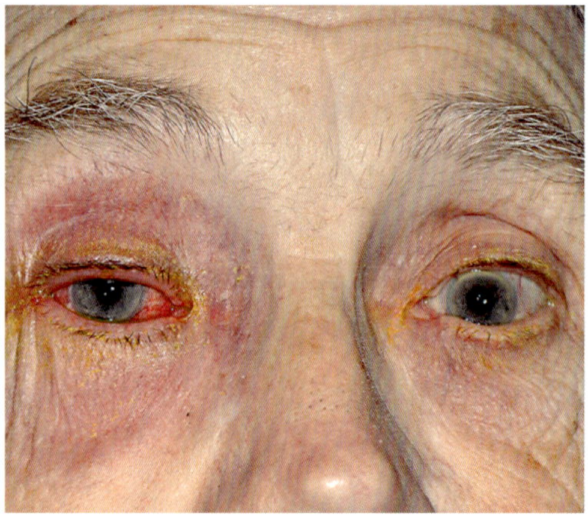

Fig. 1. Acute radiation therapy complications manifesting as periocular erythema, conjunctivitis and keratitis.

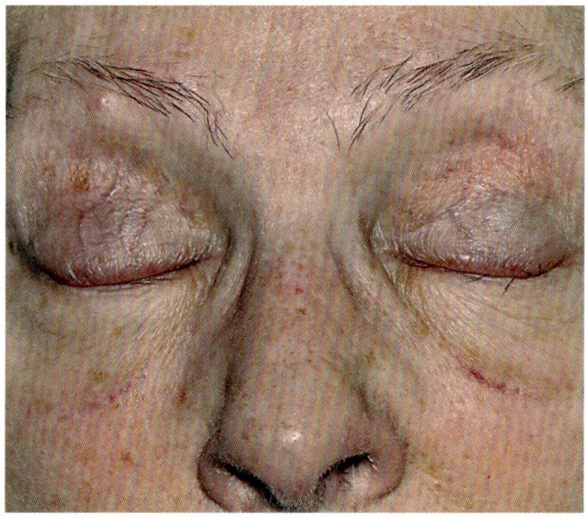

Fig. 2. Transient eyelash loss and eyelid edema 4 weeks following radiation therapy.

ma, friction, scratching or rubbing. Harsh soaps and lotions should be avoided [6]. Epiphora secondary to an eyelid abnormality may require surgical repair of ectropion or entropion with partial or full thickness grafts [7]. If a surgical approach is taken, the surgeon must consider delayed postoperative wound healing due to reduced vascularity of the irradiated tissues [3]. Epiphora may also be due to trichiasis and can effectively be managed by epilation, electrolysis, cryotherapy and argon laser ablation [3]. If the lacrimal system is involved and the patient is complaining of epiphora, nasolacrimal system intubation with silicone tubing should be considered to prevent cicatrization [7]. The tubing should be left in place for 3–9 months or until cicatrizing changes of the lid have subsided [9]. Prophylactic nasolacrimal duct intubation has been reported in patients that are at high risk [10]. If well tolerated they may be left in place longer as post radiation wound remodeling may continue even after one year. The probability of radiation effects is reduced by the use of smaller fractions, longer treatment schedules and smaller treatment volumes [11].

Adnexa

Acute

Acute complications of ocular adnexa are not common.

Late

Late effects of radiation can include orbital fat atrophy, fibrosis, ptosis, strabismus, secondary malignant tumor, growth retardation and contracture in an anophthalmic socket [4, 12, 13]. Lacrimal gland atrophy can be observed with high doses (50–60 Gy) and may cause dry eye syndrome but this is more commonly associated with radiation to the conjunctiva as discussed later in this chapter [4, 14, 15]. Radiation, particularly external beam irradiation, renders growing orbital bones in children susceptible to growth retardation (fig. 3). Marked facial deformities may occur years after doses of 40–70 Gy. Radiotherapy in children with heritable retinoblastoma increases the risk of developing a secondary malignant neoplasm [4]. Secondary malignant neoplasms may occur without the use of radiotherapy but radiation induced tumors are the most frequent. Of these, bone and soft tissue sarcomas are the most common (fig. 4) [16]. Decreasing radiation dose and delaying radiotherapy until the patient is 12 months or older has been shown to significantly decrease the risk of secondary malignant neoplasm [16–18].

Management

Treatment of dry eye is discussed in the 'Conjunctiva' section. Socket reconstruction may be required as a poorly fitting prosthesis may be the result of soft tissue atrophy, a contracted socket, and orbital hypoplasia [4]. Early recognition and, if warranted, treatment of secondary malignant neoplasm is essential.

Conjunctiva

Acute

The conjunctiva functions to protect the underlying sclera and orbit and to provide moisture to the eye. Mucin production and lacrimal duct production are essential

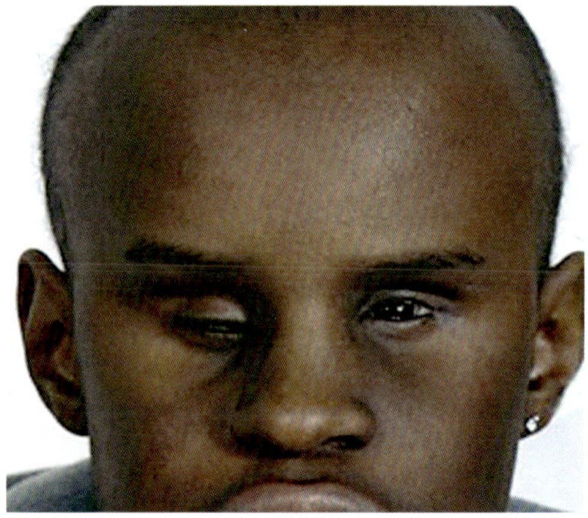

Fig. 3. Typical orbital deformity (hourglass deformity) following treatment of retinoblastoma with external radiation therapy in childhood. Additional sequelae included corneal pacification, dryness and cataracts in both eyes.

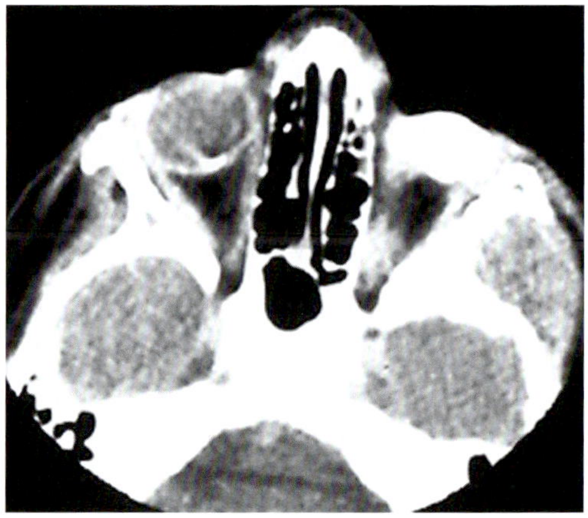

Fig. 4. A 16-year-old girl with bilateral retinoblastoma (germline mutation) treated with bilateral external radiation. On CT scan, residual calcific tumor is visible within the right globe. Prosthesis is present in the left globe. Note thickening of the sphenoid bone in the left temporal fossa (osteogenic sarcoma).

in providing integrity to the tear film and conjunctiva [19]. The conjunctiva is composed of squamous epithelium, mucin-producing goblet cells, substantia propria and the accessory lacrimal glands of Krause and Wolfring which are located in the conjunctival stroma. Acute complications of radiotherapy in the conjunctiva include conjunctivitis, chemosis, discharge and ulceration. Inflammation or conjunctivitis may be seen after one single dose of ≥5 Gy and is common in doses ≥30 Gy [1, 14, 20]. Conjunctivitis usually presents 1–3 weeks into treatment (fig. 1). Hyperemia, chemosis and a clear purulent discharge may all present simultaneously and last for a few days [1, 14]. Infection may also present as an acute complication if an ulceration of the conjunctiva is present [1].

Late

Late complications of radiotherapy include dry eye symptoms, injection, telangiectasia, subconjunctival hemorrhage, foreshortening of the fornices/symblepharon, necrosis, scaring and keratinization. Scaring and keratinization may be secondary to loss of conjunctival goblet cells. Conjunctival telangiectasia typically occur at doses exceeding 30 Gy [20]. Doses ≥35 Gy have resulted in a significant incidence of late complications of the ocular surface [20]. Keratinization, squamous metaplasia, chronic conjunctivitis and scaring of the conjunctiva can occur with doses of >50 Gy [1, 4, 7]. An increase in conjunctival epithelial stratification and a reduction of goblet cell numbers both contribute to dry eye. The tear film in these patients is usually unstable due to mucin deficiency secondary to goblet cell loss [19, 21]. Although decreased mucin production may be an important factor in dry eye, radiation can also affect the meibomian glands and accessory lacrimal glands, and, therefore, all layers of the tear film can be affected [7]. Recurrent corneal erosions from recurrent mechanical abrasion or erosion caused by the palpebral conjunctiva may progress to ulceration and infection leading to opacification and/or perforation [7]. Symblepharon is frequent with doses of above 80–100 Gy and may lead to exposure keratopathy and limited ocular motility [14, 22]. Necrosis may occur in patients after brachytherapy with doses to the conjunctiva of 90–300 Gy [1]. Subconjunctival hemorrhages are rare and usually self-limited.

Management

A lubricating ointment may be used liberally to preserve and replace moisture from the lost or damaged goblet cells and keratinization [1]. Topical corticosteroids may be beneficial in the setting of injection and chemosis but should be used cautiously because of side effects that include cataracts and glaucoma. Vitamin A ophthalmic ointment (tretinoin 0.01 or 0.1%) may reverse squamous metaplasia and loss of vascularization from scar formation [19, 23, 24]. Amniotic membrane transplantation may be used to reconstruct conjunctival defects after resection, after symblepharon lysis or immunomodulation of the inflammatory response in severe cases [25]. By reducing the dose build-up on the conjunctival surface, the risk of conjunctival toxicity can be reduced by treating with the eye open when megavoltage radiotherapy is delivered [3].

Cornea

Acute

Most acute corneal injury to the cornea is secondary to loss of the tear film and not to direct injury to the cornea (fig. 1) [3]. The epithelium is the most anterior surface and has the ability to regenerate without scarring. The stroma will also regenerate, but with scarring. The endothelium does not regenerate and is affected with radiation doses of 10–20 Gy [1]. Early effects are common and include epithelial defects, inflammation (keratitis) and hypoesthesia [26]. Patients may complain of a foreign body sensation and epiphora [1]. Punctate epithelial keratitis is commonly seen on microscopic examination with conventionally fractionated doses of 30–50 Gy [27]. They are best seen with fluorescein staining and a cobalt blue filter from a slit lamp microscope [1]. Corneal edema may be seen with doses of 40–50 Gy [27]. Keratoconjunctivitis occurs especially when doses of more than 50 Gy are used to treat the eye. In these cases the patient may complain of photophobia as well as foreign body sensation and epiphora [8]. Corneal ulceration may occur in patients who received >60 Gy and has been reported with 20 Gy delivered in a single dose [27].

Late

Late complications include epithelial desquamation, corneal neovascularization, corneal edema, corneal melting/perforation, keratinization, dry eye and corneal hypoesthesia [1, 4, 14, 22]. Corneal hypoesthesia may be present as both an acute or a late complication. Corneal desquamation may persist for months as these radiated corneal epithelial cells have a poor capacity to heal [8]. These erosions may progress to ulcerations and ultimately to perforation and are typically complicated by a neurotrophic component that usually occurs months after treatment [1]. Ulcerations are common when doses of ≥40 Gy are used [14]. Changes in the conjunctiva and tear film may eventually manifest in the cornea as diffuse punctate epithelial erosions to corneal ulcers or even perforation. Keratinization and scarring are seen when doses of ≥50 Gy are used [8]. Corneal decompensation secondary to stem cell loss may also be seen [7]. The incidence of lacrimal gland fibrosis and atrophy with subsequent keratitis sicca sharply increases with doses ≥50 Gy. Corneal neovascularization and subsequent opacification is frequently present within 9–10 months when doses ≥57 Gy are used [28]. A dose-dependent curve has been reported for dry eye with minimal risk at doses <30 Gy that steeply increases at doses >40 and reaching 100% rate of severe dry eye with doses >57 Gy [3, 29].

Management

Management of keratitis consists of aggressive lubrication and antibiotic drops as necessary [7]. Aggressive lubrication either with drops or lubricating ointment may be performed liberally by the patient to help with symptoms [7, 28]. Preservative-free solutions are recommended if dosing that is more frequent than 4–6 times a day as the preservative may cause epithelial toxicity. Moisture chamber goggles improve humidity and decrease evaporation and may be used at night. Another approach is to slow down tear drainage with punctual occlusion either temporal with punctual plugs or permanent with punctual cautery [7]. Patients should be encouraged to avoid fans, wind, smoke and dry air conditions that contribute to corneal dryness. Management of recurrent corneal erosions should be targeted at the underlying pathology. The upper eyelid should be everted and the clinician should look for any changes in the palpebral conjunctiva (metaplastic conjunctiva) that might be causing the epithelial defect. Lid positioning and closure should be assessed and repaired if necessary. Cultures, tarsorrhaphy, punctual occlusion, aggressive lubrication and topical antibiotic therapy should be considered for infected corneal ulcers [7]. Bandage contact lenses have been used to promote corneal healing in patients with severe radiation-induced keratitis [1, 30]. Hypertonic saline solution may also be used in the setting of recurrent corneal erosions or corneal edema. Amniotic membrane transplantation may be used to promote corneal healing [25, 31].

Corneal glue or keratoplasty may be required in the cases of pending or apparent corneal perforation [1].

Episclera and Sclera

Acute

The sclera and episclera may become injected 2–4 weeks after radiation treatment. Resolution is usually spontaneous and requires no treatment [1].

Late

Thinning, melting and atrophy occur several years after doses of 20–30 Gy are administered [1]. Necrosis has been reported after brachytherapy and scleral perforation although rare, can also occur [14].

Management

Management of scleral thinning is aimed at maintaining the integrity of the globe [7]. It appears as a blue-grayish or black coloration of the sclera on gross examination. Care must be taken as pigmented episcleral deposits following ruthenium or iodine plaque brachytherapy have been described and may mimic thinning or extra scleral extension of a melanocytic lesion (fig. 5) [32]. These deposits appeared between 1 and 6 months after treatment were 8 μm to 3 mm in size and increased in

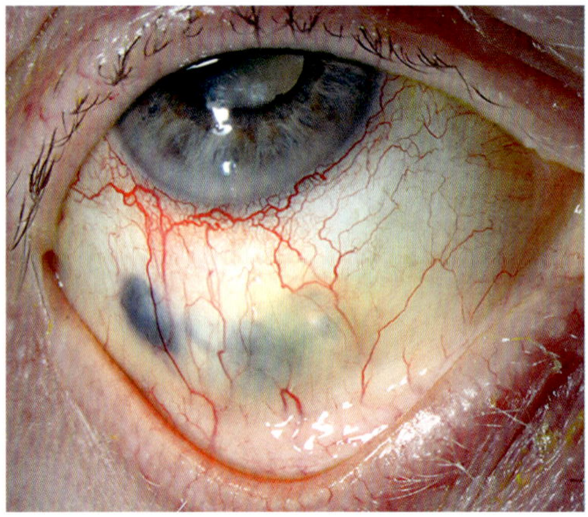

Fig. 5. Scleral atrophy 10 months following plaque radiotherapy for a large ciliochoroidal melanoma. Note subepithelial pigment migration that mimics extrascleral extension of the melanoma.

numbers until 7 years after treatment. Thinning of more than 50% may require a conjunctival graft to cover the defect. In more severe cases, a scleral or periosteal graft may be needed [7].

Iris

Acute

The iris is relatively radiation resistant [3]. Severe persistent iritis has been observed after fractionated doses of ≥60–70 Gy or a single dose of ≥10 Gy [1, 3]. Patients may complain of pain, photophobia, red eye and blurry vision [14].

Late

Rubeosis iridis and neovascular glaucoma are late complications that follow exposure to high radiation doses. Rubeosis iridis occurs in 4–25% of cases treated with iodine-125 plaque brachytherapy at a mean of 26.7 months [26]. Rates as high as 62% have been reported 5 years after treatment of eyes with large choroidal melanomas treated with iodine-125 brachytherapy [33]. Abnormal fibrovascularization of the angle and subsequent closure of the outflow channels may lead to subsequent neovascular glaucoma and may be present in up to 20% of eyes treated with radiotherapy [3]. Neovascularization is almost always ischemic but may be due to untreated choroidal melanoma, ischemia associated with radiation retinopathy or ischemia from radiation damage to the iris [chapter by Seregard et al., this vol.; 26]. Risk factors for the development of glaucoma include higher radiation doses, diabetes, vitreous hemorrhage and retinal detachment [34]. In plaque brachytherapy induced cases, studies using isotopes other than iodine-125 such as cobalt-60 and palladium-103, location anterior tumor, greater tumor size and height and desinsertion of a lateral muscle have all been associated with higher rates of neovascularization [26, 33, 35]. The patient may present with rapid loss of vision, severe pain and headache [7]. Iris atrophy is usually seen more than 3 years after treatment with high doses that are uncommonly used today [14].

Management

Primary management of iritis includes cycloplegic drops and topical steroids. Gonioscopy as well as a thorough exam of the iris and anterior chamber prior to dilation are essential for early detection. Laser pan retinal photocoagulation is sometimes effective in inducing regression of the iris/angle neovascularization [3]. Administration of intravitreal anti-VEGF mass adjunctive therapy may be beneficial [36]. Intraocular pressure should be managed medically when possible yet glaucoma secondary to peripheral anterior synechia or angle closure will unlikely respond to these treatments and if refractory to medical treatment may require surgical intervention.

Lens

Acute

Transient myopia has been reported within weeks after radiotherapy [1].

Late

The crystalline lens is the most radiosensitive organ and doses of less than 2 Gy have been reported to cause cataracts [37]. The incidence of cataracts after radiation exposure is high with a wide range of incidence reported, between 45 and 100% [2]. The formation of cataracts may occur as early as 1 month following treatment and as late as 7 years depending upon several factors including the type of radiation, total dose, delivery portals and the time after exposure [38]. Ionizing radiation has been primarily associated with posterior subcapsular cataracts although cortical and nuclear changes have also been reported [38]. The association between cataracts and corticosteroids has been well documented and may play a role in cataract formation in patients who receive radiotherapy as most of them also receive corticosteroids.

Management

Cataract removal is the only curative treatment for radiation-induced cataracts. Special considerations must be taken by the surgeon as these patients might have other radiation-induced changes in their anterior chamber that can make cataract removal more challenging. Prevention with lens-sparing radiation techniques is helpful in preventing or delaying cataract formation. The use of lead shields and fractionation of the radiation dose has been shown to decrease the total dose of radiation to the lens [1, 39].

References

1 Servodidio CA, Abramson DH: Acute and long-term effects of radiation therapy to the eye in children. Cancer Nurs 1993;16:371–381.

2 Ferrufino-Ponce ZK, Henderson BA: Radiotherapy and cataract formation. Semin Ophthalmol 2006;21:171–180.

3 Jeganathan VS, Wirth A, MacManus MP: Ocular risks from orbital and periorbital radiation therapy: a critical review. Int J Radiat Oncol Biol Phys 2011;79:650–659.

4 Taban M, Taban M, Bolling J, Singh AD: Ocular complications of radiotherapy; in Singh AD, Damato BE, Pe'er J, Murphree AL, Perry JD (eds): Clinical Ophthalmic Oncology, ed 1. Philadelphia, Saunders-Elsevier, 2007, pp 45–49.

5 Finger PT: Radiation therapy for choroidal melanoma. Surv Ophthalmol 1997;42:215–232.

6 Walker VA: Skin care during radiotherapy. Nurs Times 1982;78:2068–2070.

7 Gordon KB, Char DH, Sagerman RH: Late effects of radiation on the eye and ocular adnexa. Int J Radiat Oncol Biol Phys 1995;31:1123–1139.

8 Haik BG, Jereb B, Abramson DH, Ellsworth RM: Ophthalmic Radiotherapy. New York, Churchill-Livingstone, 1983.

9 Lovato AA, Char DH, Castro JR, Kroll SM: The effect of silicone nasolacrimal intubation on epiphora after helium ion irradiation of uveal melanomas. Am J Ophthalmol 1989;108:431–434.

10 de Smet MD, Buffam FV, Fairey RN, Voss NJ: Prevention of radiation-induced stenosis of the nasolacrimal duct. Can J Ophthalmol 1990;25:145–147.

11 Bentzen SM, Thames HD: A 100-year Nordic perspective on the dose-time problem in radiobiology. Acta Oncol 1995;34:1031–1040.

12 Heyn R, Ragab A, Raney RB Jr, Ruymann F, Tefft M, Lawrence W Jr, et al: Late effects of therapy in orbital rhabdomyosarcoma in children. A report from the Intergroup Rhabdomyosarcoma Study. Cancer 1986;57:1738–1743.

13 Larson DL, Kroll S, Jaffe N, Serure A, Goepfert H: Long-term effects of radiotherapy in childhood and adolescence. Am J Surg 1990;160:348–351.

14 Brady LW, Shields J, Augusburger J, Markoe A, Karlsson UL: Complications from radiation therapy to the eye. Front Radiat Ther Oncol 1989;23:238–250.

15 Parsons JT, Fitzgerald CR, Hood CI, Ellingwood KE, Bova FJ, Million RR: The effects of irradiation on the eye and optic nerve. Int J Radiat Oncol Biol Phys 1983;9:609–622.

16 Merchant T: Teletherapy: indications, risks and new delivery options; in Singh A, Damato B, Pe'er J, Murphree A, Perry J (eds): Essentials in Ophthalmic Oncology. Thorofare, SLACK Incorporated, 2006, pp 462–467.

17 Abramson DH, Frank CM: Second nonocular tumors in survivors of bilateral retinoblastoma: a possible age effect on radiation-related risk. Ophthalmology 1998;105:573–579.

18 Moll AC, Imhof SM, Schouten-Van Meeteren AY, Kuik DJ, Hofman P, Boers M: Second primary tumors in hereditary retinoblastoma: a register-based study, 1945–1997: is there an age effect on radiation-related risk? Ophthalmology 2001;108:1109–1114.

19 Tseng SC: Topical tretinoin treatment for severe dry-eye disorders. J Am Acad Dermatol 1986;15:860–866.

20 Stafford SL, Kozelsky TF, Garrity JA, Kurtin PJ, Leavitt JA, Martenson JA, et al: Orbital lymphoma: radiotherapy outcome and complications. Radiother Oncol 2001;59:139–144.

21 Heimann H, Coupland SE, Gochman R, Hellmich M, Foerster MH: Alterations in expression of mucin, tenascin-C and syndecan-1 in the conjunctiva following retinal surgery and plaque radiotherapy. Graefes Arch Clin Exp Ophthalmol 2001;239:488–495.

22 Hempel M, Hinkelbein W: Eye sequelae following external irradiation. Rec Results Cancer Res 1993;130:231–236.

23 Carlier C, Coste J, Etchepare M, Amedee-Manesme O: Conjunctival impression cytology with transfer as a field-applicable indicator of vitamin A status for mass screening. Int J Epidemiol 1992;21:373–380.
24 Soong HK, Martin NF, Wagoner MD, Alfonso E, Mandelbaum SH, Laibson PR, et al: Topical retinoid therapy for squamous metaplasia of various ocular surface disorders. A multicenter, placebo-controlled double-masked study. Ophthalmology 1988;95: 1442–1446.
25 Chen HJ, Pires RT, Tseng SC: Amniotic membrane transplantation for severe neurotrophic corneal ulcers. Br J Ophthalmol 2000;84:826–833.
26 Wen JC, Oliver SC, McCannel TA: Ocular complications following I-125 brachytherapy for choroidal melanoma. Eye (Lond) 2009;23:1254–1268.
27 Barabino S, Raghavan A, Loeffler J, Dana R: Radiotherapy-induced ocular surface disease. Cornea 2005; 24:909–914.
28 Durkin SR, Roos D, Higgs B, Casson RJ, Selva D: Ophthalmic and adnexal complications of radiotherapy. Acta Ophthalmol Scand 2007;85:240–250.
29 Bessell EM, Henk JM, Whitelocke RA, Wright JE: Ocular morbidity after radiotherapy of orbital and conjunctival lymphoma. Eye (Lond) 1987;1:90–96.
30 Ingraham HJ, Perry HD, Donnenfeld ED, Epstein AB: Glued-on, rigid gas-permeable contact lens for severe radiation-induced keratitis. Am J Ophthalmol 1992;113:538–540.
31 Azuara-Blanco A, Pillai CT, Dua HS: Amniotic membrane transplantation for ocular surface reconstruction. Br J Ophthalmol 1999;83:399–402.
32 Toivonen P, Kivela T: Pigmented episcleral deposits after brachytherapy of uveal melanoma. Ophthalmology 2006;113:865–873.
33 Puusaari I, Heikkonen J, Kivela T: Ocular complications after iodine brachytherapy for large uveal melanomas. Ophthalmology 2004;111:1768–1777.
34 Daftari IK, Char DH, Verhey LJ, Castro JR, Petti PL, Meecham WJ, et al: Anterior segment sparing to reduce charged particle radiotherapy complications in uveal melanoma. Int J Radiat Oncol Biol Phys 1997; 39:997–1010.
35 Detorakis ET, Engstrom RE Jr, Wallace R, Straatsma BR: Iris and anterior chamber angle neovascularization after iodine-125 brachytherapy for uveal melanoma. Ophthalmology 2005;112:505–510.
36 Douat J, Auriol S, Mahieu-Durringer L, Ancele E, Pagot-Mathis V, Mathis A: Intravitreal bevacizumab for treatment of neovascular glaucoma. Report of 20 cases. J Fr Ophtalmol 2009;32:652–663.
37 Hoehn ME, Irshad F, Kerr NC, Wilson MW: Outcomes after cataract extraction in young children with radiation-induced cataracts and retinoblastoma. J AAPOS 2010;14:232–234.
38 Cogan DG, Donaldson DD, Reese AB: Clinical and pathological characteristics of radiation cataract. AMA Arch Ophthalmol 1952;47:55–70.
39 Esik O, Ikeda H, Mukai K, Kaneko A: A retrospective analysis of different modalities for treatment of primary orbital non-Hodgkin's lymphomas. Radiother Oncol 1996;38:13–18.

Arun D. Singh, MD
Director, Department of Ophthalmic Oncology, Cole Eye Institute
Cleveland Clinic Foundation, 9500 Euclid Avenue
Cleveland, OH 44195 (USA)
E-Mail singha@ccf.org

Singh AD, Pelayes DE, Seregard S, Macklis R (eds): Ophthalmic Radiation Therapy. Techniques and Applications.
Dev Ophthalmol. Basel, Karger, 2013, vol 52, pp 114–123 (DOI: 10.1159/000351088)

Radiation Therapy: Posterior Segment Complications

Stefan Seregard[a] · David E. Pelayes[b, c] · Arun D. Singh[d]

[a]St Eriks Eye Hospital, Karoliniska Institutet, Stockholm, Sweden; [b]Department of Ophthalmology, Maimonides University, and [c]Department of Ophthalmology, Buenos Aires University, Buenos Aires, Argentina; [d]Department of Ophthalmic Oncology, Cole Eye Institute, Cleveland Clinic Foundation, Cleveland, Ohio, USA

Abstract

Therapeutic radiation to the posterior segment of the eye is a common option for posterior segment tumors. Such tumors are often malignant, but sometimes, benign neoplasms are treated with ionizing radiation. Also, non-neoplastic intraocular lesions like wet age-related macular degeneration may be treated with radiotherapy. Orbital disease, both neoplastic lesions like optic nerve sheath meningioma and non-neoplastic entities like Graves' ophthalmopathy may be treated with radiotherapy and this may include radiation of the optic nerve and posterior segment of the eye. Occasionally, radiotherapy of extraocular malignant disease, involving, e.g. the paranasal sinuses, may cause significant radiation damage to the eye. Complications after radiation to the posterior segment of the eye are largely related to the radiation dose to the posterior segment. The amount of irradiated volume of normal tissue and fractionation are also important for the development of radiation complications to the posterior segment. Radiation retinopathy is the most common complication of the posterior segment, but radiation optic neuropathy also occurs frequently. Radiation scleral necrosis is less frequent probably due to the radioresistance of the scleral collagen. These complications have the potential to cause blindness (radiation retinopathy and optic neuropathy) or enucleation of the eye (scleral necrosis). Although numerous treatments have been advocated, management of radiation-induced damage remains controversial. Efficacy for any treatment still needs to be proven and, if possible, the best option by far is to minimize radiation changes to normal tissue.

Radiation Retinopathy

Radiation retinopathy is a chronic and progressive vasculopathy of the retinal capillaries primarily caused by endothelial damage to the vessel walls after radiotherapy. This damage causes capillary dilation, increased vascular permeability, endothelial sloughing, thrombosis, retinal cotton wool spots, retinal exudates and hemorrhages.

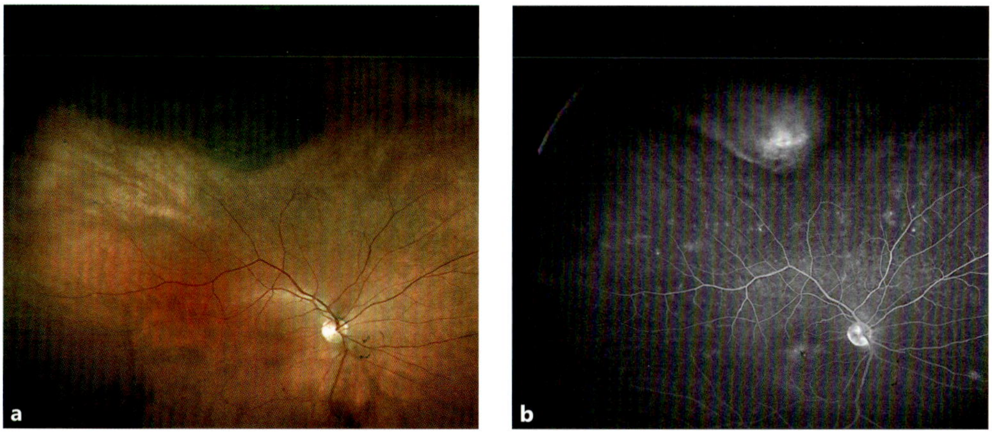

Fig. 1. Fundus photograph (**a**) and fluorescein angiography (**b**) showing peripheral capillary nonperfusion.

Later loss of pericytes as well as endothelial cells results in capillary drop-out and full-thickness retinal atrophy. By fluorescein angiography, capillary nonperfusion is evident and this remains the gold standard to demonstrate radiation retinopathy (fig. 1) [1–3]. Presence of capillary nonperfusion strongly suggests that retinal ischemia is involved in the development of radiation retinopathy. Interestingly, some features presumed to indicate early retinopathy (e.g. microaneurysms) is present in a subset of patients well before radiotherapy is initiated [4]. This questions the specificity of some retinal findings apart from capillary nonperfusion.

Radiation retinopathy is present in 42% at 5 years after brachytherapy for posterior uveal melanoma [2], and two thirds of patients with radiation-induced retinopathy will eventually develop proliferative retinopathy [5]. Although radiation retinopathy may arise early, presentation is often delayed and occurs from 6 months to 5 years after radiotherapy with a peak at 1–2 years after treatment [2]. The first finding of radiation retinopathy may be reduced visual acuity due to subclinical macular edema. There is some evidence that macular edema detected by optical coherence tomography predicts later development of clinically evident radiation maculopathy by an average of 5 months, although maculopathy is not always preceded by subclinical macular edema (fig. 2) [6].

The frequency of radiation retinopathy is related to the total radiotherapy dose, fractionation (if any) and retinal volume irradiated. Radiation retinopathy should be separated from tumor necrosis with secondary retinal exudation. When the macula is involved, radiation retinopathy is often referred to as radiation maculopathy. Proliferative radiation retinopathy may follow from ischemic radiation retinopathy. Retinopathy is seen in up to 60% of patients with brachytherapy for choroidal melanoma and less frequently in intraocular tumors that receive a lower dose, e.g. retinoblastoma, metastases, choroidal hemangioma. Radiation retinopathy may also develop after

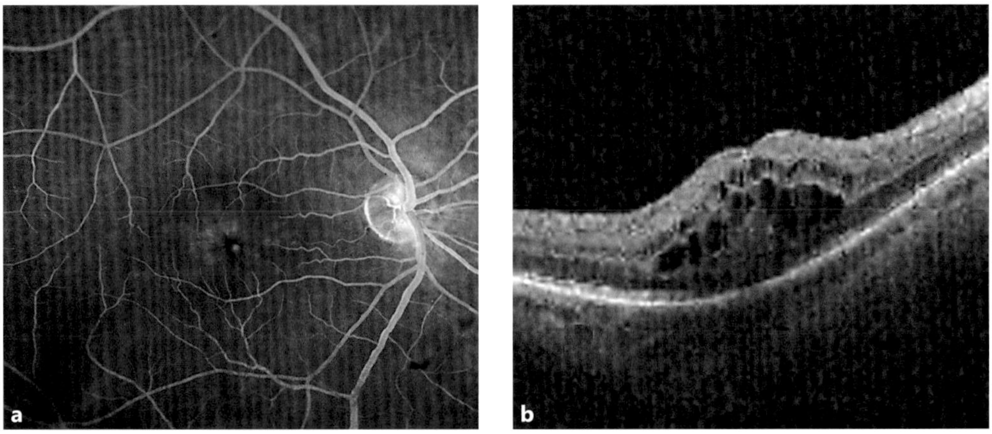

Fig. 2. Radiation induced macular edema, appearance on fluorescein angiography (**a**) and by optical coherence tomography (**b**).

radiotherapy for extraocular tumors, when the field includes all or part of the retina, e.g. tumors of the paranasal sinuses or optic nerve.

Although radiation retinopathy was initially reported after external beam radiotherapy, it is now mostly seen after brachytherapy [2]. Eventually, more than half of patients receiving 65 Gy to healthy retina will develop radiation retinopathy [7]. It is generally believed that radiation retinopathy rarely occurs when the dose to healthy retina is less than 35 Gy, although retinopathy has been reported after doses as low as 16 Gy [8]. Charged particle irradiation may cause radiation retinopathy in 8–15% of patients after doses as low as 16–20 CGE in 2–4 fractions [9, 10]. Moreover, a few patients developed radiation retinopathy after low-dose epimacular strontium-90 brachytherapy (24 Gy) for wet age-related macular degeneration [11]. Pre-existing retinal vascular disease, like diabetic retinopathy, predisposes for more frequent and aggressive radiation retinopathy.

Proliferative radiation retinopathy may develop from ischemic radiation retinopathy (fig. 3). The median time from plaque radiotherapy to presentation of proliferative radiation retinopathy is 2.5 years and up to 80% of patients with this form of radiation retinopathy will develop vitreous hemorrhage [12]. The incidence of proliferative radiation retinopathy is related to tumor size and hence to the radiotherapy dose to healthy retina; 25% of patients treated with plaque radiotherapy for tumors larger than 8 mm in height develop neovascular retinopathy [13].

Occasionally, exudative retinal detachment leading to a bullous detachment occurs shortly after plaque radiotherapy, in particular when plaques with a high dose rate are used (fig. 4). This retinal detachment usually resolves over a period of months or years. Extensive radiation retinopathy may lead to retinal detachment. Although retinal photoreceptors are fairly radioresistant, retinal atrophy may develop after long-standing retinal detachment or macular edema (fig. 5) [14].

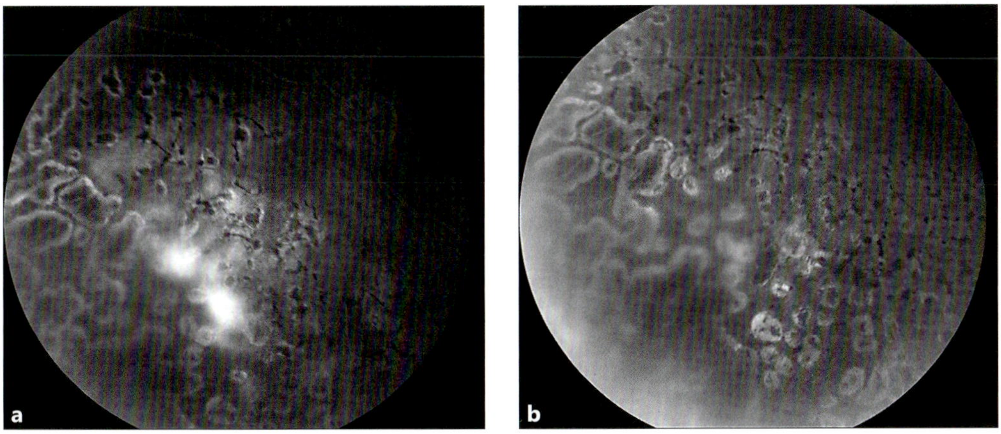

Fig. 3. Proliferative radiation retinopathy. **a** Fluorescein angiography showing leakage due to retinal neovascularization. One week after treatment with intravitreal bevacizumab (in addition to prior pan retinal photocoagulation). **b** Angiography of the same region without any leakage.

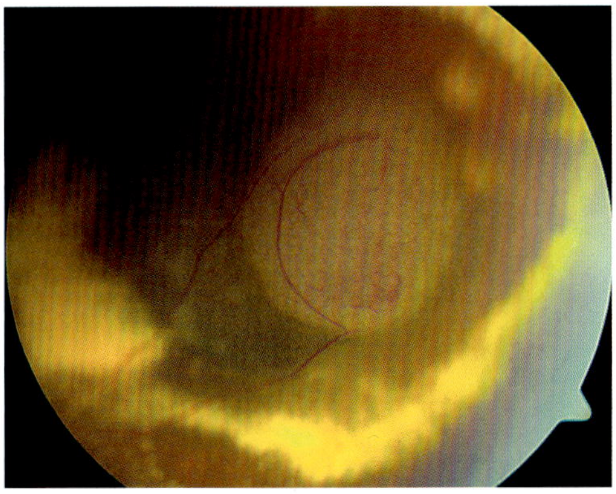

Fig. 4. Exudative retinal detachment due to extensive lipid and serous exudation from treated melanoma.

Theoretically, fractionation may reduce the risk for radiation retinopathy, but 60% of patients exposed to stereotactic photon radiotherapy using 60 Gy in 5 fractions will have radiation maculopathy at 5 years [15]. Moreover, radiation maculopathy develops in 90% of patients treated with proton beam radiotherapy for uveal melanoma (70 CGE in 5 fractions) [16]. Even a few (1%) of the patients with Graves' ophthalmopathy treated with low-dose external beam radiotherapy (20 Gy in 10 fractions) to the orbit including most of the posterior segment will develop some radiation retinopathy [17, 18].

A wide range of treatments have been used for radiation retinopathy. These techniques include panretinal or focal laser photocoagulation, photodynamic therapy, intravitreal or periocular triamcinolone, oral pentoxifylline, hyperbaric oxygen, intravitreal anti-VEGF agents, and recently intravitreal silicone oil placement prior to brachy-

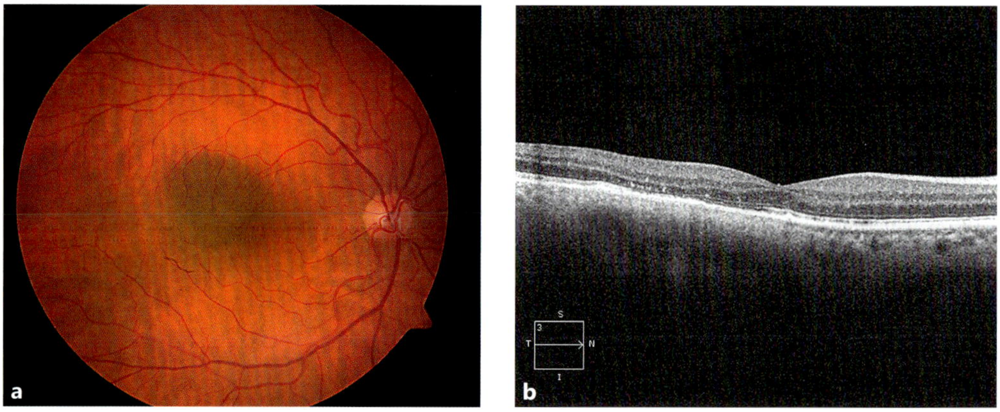

Fig. 5. Retinal photoreceptor and retinal atrophy as a manifestation of radiation retinopathy. **a** Fundus appearance after treatment of a small choroidal melanoma. **b** Optical coherence tomography reveals disruption of photoreceptor IS/OS junction line.

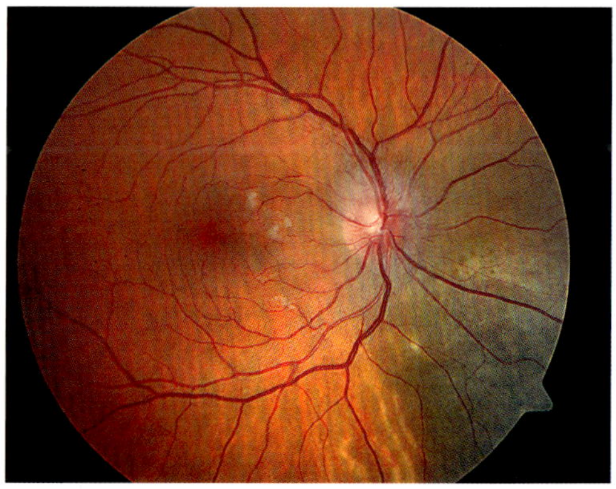

Fig. 6. Radiation-induced optic neuropathy typically presents as disc edema and hemorrhages at the optic nerve head. Note associated cotton wool spots.

therapy in an attempt to attenuate scatter radiation [19–21]. Although a few randomized clinical trials are currently being planned or pursued, none of the treatments above have yet proven their value for radiation retinopathy [21]. Reducing radiation exposure to the macula by the careful choice of radionuclide and eccentric plaque fixation when possible remains the best choice to minimize visual complications.

Radiation Optic Neuropathy

Radiation-induced optic neuropathy typically presents with painless and rapid visual loss occurring months to years after radiation to the optic nerve [22]. Findings may include disc edema and hemorrhages at the optic nerve head (so-called papillopathy) (fig. 6).

When only the postlaminar optic nerve is involved, the clinical appearance is usually more subtle with progressive pallor of the optic nerve head [1, 23]. The pathogenesis is believed to include vascular occlusion with secondary axonal death, primary radiation-induced axonal necrosis or a combination of these [23].

The damage to the optic nerve is related to the total dose, volume of optic nerve irradiated and fractionation. Previously, exposure to 50 Gy in a single dose was regarded as a safe upper limit to avoid optic neuropathy [24]. More recent data, however, indicate that a single dose of less than 12 Gy will induce radiation optic neuropathy in 1% of patients [25]. Data also suggest that no patient receiving less than 8 Gy to the anterior optic pathways will develop optic neuropathy, but the frequency then rises steeply to 78% when the dose is 15 Gy or more following stereotactic radiosurgery [26]. Episcleral brachytherapy of posterior segment tumors typically irradiates a smaller portion of the optic nerve than stereotactic radiosurgery. Nonetheless, patients with juxtapapillary uveal melanoma or large uveal melanoma away from the optic disc managed by iodine brachytherapy will receive a large dose to the optic nerve head (median 69 Gy) and half of these patients will develop radiation optic neuropathy [27, 28].

Fractionation significantly reduces radiation toxicity and for doses at <1.8 Gy per fraction, radiation damage increases markedly first when the total dose is more than 60 Gy. A similar increase in radiation toxicity is evident for single doses above 12 Gy [22]. External beam radiotherapy (20 Gy in 10 fractions) to the orbit for Graves' ophthalmopathy usually fails to generate radiation optic neuropathy [18], but there are exceptions [29]. Proton beam radiotherapy is typically delivered in 5 fractions during a period of 7–10 days. For parapapillary choroidal melanoma within 1.5 disc diameters of the optic nerve head, the standard dose to the optic nerve is 50–70 CGE and approximately two thirds of these patients will develop radiation papillopathy after a median of 2 years [30]. Apparently, the advantage of fractionation needs to be balanced against the larger volume of normal tissue irradiated when using external beam radiotherapy. Although stereotactic radiotherapy for juxtapapillary uveal melanoma characteristically uses 70 Gy delivered in 5 fractions, data suggest that the 50-month actuarial rate of optic papillopathy is 39 and 74% following iodine brachytherapy and stereotactic radiotherapy, respectively [31]. This lower complication rate for brachytherapy may be related to a volumetric effect.

The clinical course of radiation optic neuropathy differs from that of radiation retinopathy as there is some scope for spontaneous improvement of vision after optic nerve damage. Notably, almost one third of patients who develop radiation papillopathy after proton beam radiotherapy for juxtapapillary uveal melanoma will experience significant spontaneous improvement during the first 5 years after therapy [30]. It seems that radiation damage is more likely to occur with increasing age [32, 33].

There is anecdotal evidence to suggest some benefit for a number of treatments for radiation-induced optic neuropathy. These include systemic corticosteroids, hyperbaric oxygen therapy and anticoagulation, but there is no proven efficacy for any of these treatments [23, 34]. Techniques to minimize radiation exposure and hence collateral damage to the optic nerve include the use of collimated plaques for iodine brachytherapy, and improved dose modulation and fractionation for external beam radiotherapy.

Radiation Scleral Necrosis

Radiation scleral necrosis is a rare complication typically seen in large uveal melanoma treated with brachytherapy including a high scleral dose. The collagen fibers of the sclera gradually dissolve leaving a thinned, translucent layer. Necrosis is often partial but may progress to full thickness melting with ocular perforation if left untreated. In most cases, however, scleral thinning is stabilized leaving the regressed tumor covered by a thin scleral lamella, some episcleral tissue and conjunctiva. The safe maximum radiotherapy dose to the sclera to avoid scleral melting is not known. Although scleral necrosis occasionally may present as early as 1 month after plaque radiotherapy [35, 36], onset is typically delayed for at least 1 year and sometimes even up to 10 years after radiation therapy [37]. This time delay and quiet mode of presentation sometimes causes radiation scleromalacia to be confused with local tumor recurrence.

The pathogenetic mechanisms leading to radiation scleral necrosis are largely unknown although radiation damage to the scleral blood supply leading to scleral ischemia has been implicated [5]. Additionally, there has been speculation in early-onset cases of a possible inadvertent ocular perforation or muscle disinsertion during surgery leading to scleral ischemia or the presence of occult autoimmune vasculitis [35].

Charged particle irradiation of intraocular tumors allows for a comparatively moderate scleral dose (typically 60 CGE) and radiotherapy necrosis arises in approximately 0.5% or less [37]. Episcleral brachytherapy necessarily includes a higher dose to the sclera, and scleromalacia requiring a patch scleral graft a few years after palladium brachytherapy may occur after doses of 200 Gy to the inner sclera [38]. The incidence of radiation scleral necrosis ranges from <1% in small and medium-sized tumors to 7% in large uveal melanoma (>8 mm in height) treated by iodine brachytherapy [13, 37]. Scleral necrosis appears to be more frequent in ciliary body melanoma and occurs in 11% of eyes at 5 years after brachytherapy. Here, scleral necrosis is associated with high intraocular pressure (>20 mm Hg) and tumors thicker than 6–7 mm [36, 39]. This suggests that scleral melting may be related to a mechanical effect of high intraocular pressure or simply that the radiotherapy dose was excessive [39]. Interestingly, a small extraocular extension in uveal melanoma does not seem to be associated with scleral necrosis, possibly because scleral integrity is not compromised as most tumor cells follow a scleral emissary [40].

Ruthenium-106 has a threefold faster dose fall-off than iodine-125 and typically the highest scleral doses are seen in patients with thick uveal melanoma managed by ruthenium brachytherapy. Approximately 20% of patients receiving a median of

1,000 Gy to the tumor base (with an even higher dose to the sclera) may develop scleral necrosis [41]. Conversely, Bergman et al. [42] provided a scleral surface dose of 1,000–1,500 Gy in 85 patients and >1,500 Gy in 23 patients treated with ruthenium-106 for thick posterior uveal melanoma. Only 1 of these patients had scleral necrosis.

Most cases of radiation-induced scleral necrosis stabilize and need only to be observed. When progression is evident a scleral patch graft may be necessary to maintain scleral integrity. Care should be taken to harvest a graft large enough to suture it to healthy sclera away from the area of necrosis. Eventually, enucleation of the eye may be required for some cases with ocular perforation or near full thickness scleral necrosis.

Conclusion

Radiation damage to the posterior segment may follow any form of radiotherapy. Typically, radiation-induced lesions appear several months or even years after radiotherapy, but acute complications may occur. Some complications like radiation retinopathy are frequent, and some like radiation scleral necrosis are distinctly uncommon. Traditionally, 35 and 50 Gy have been regarded as the safe upper limits to not develop retinopathy and optic neuropathy, respectively. In fact, there is much evidence that radiation damage may frequently develop following exposure to much lower doses and there appears to be no safe upper limit. Management of radiation-induced damage is challenging and response to treatment is at best transient. Better dose modulation in the future will hopefully minimize exposure of healthy tissue to high doses of ionizing radiation and prevent radiation-induced collateral damage.

References

1 Brown GC, Shields JA, Sanborn G, Augsburger JJ, Savino PJ, Schatz NJ: Radiation retinopathy. Ophthalmology 1982;89:1494–1501.

2 Gündüz K, Shields CL, Shields JA, Cater J, Freire JE, Brady LW: Radiation retinopathy following plaque radiotherapy for posterior uveal melanoma. Arch Ophthalmol 1999;117:609–614.

3 Horgan N, Shields CL, Mashayekhi A, Shields JA: Classification and treatment of radiation maculopathy. Curr Opin Ophthalmol 2010;21:233–238.

4 Boldt CH, Melia BM, Liu JC, Reynolds SM: I-125 brachytherapy for choroidal melanoma. Photographic and angiographic abnormalities: the Collaborative Ocular Melanoma Study: COMS report No. 30. Ophthalmology 2009;116:106–115.

5 Shields CL, Shields JA, Cater J, Othmane I, Singh AD, Micaily B: Plaque radiotherapy for retinoblastoma. Long-term control and treatment complications in 208 tumors. Ophthalmology 2001;108:2116–2121.

6 Horgan N, Shields CL, Mashayekhi A, Teixeira LF, Materin M, Shields JA: Early macular morphological changes following plaque radiotherapy for uveal melanoma. Retina 2008;28:263–273.

7 Emami B, Lyman J, Brown A, Cola L, Goitein M, Munzenrider JE, Shank B, Solin LJ, Wesson M: Tolerance of normal tissue to therapeutic irradiation. Int J Radiat Oncolol Phys 1991;21:109–122.

8 Elsås T, Thorud E, Jetne V, Conradi IS: Retinopathy after low dose irradiation for an intracranial tumor of the frontal lobe. A case report. Acta Ophthalmol (Copenh) 1988;66:65–68.

9 Zambarakji HJ, Lane AM, Erzra E, Gauthier D, Goitein, Adamds JA, Munzenrider JE, Miller JW, Gragoudas ES: Proton beam irradiation for neovascular age-related macular degeneration. Ophthalmology 2006;113:2012–2019.
10 Levy-Gabriel C, Lumbroso-Le Rouic L, Plancher C, Rendale D, Delacroix S, Asslain B, Habrand J-L, Desjardins L: Long-term results of low dose proton beam therapy for circumscribed choroidal hemangioma. Retina 2009;29:170–175.
11 Dugel PU, Bebchuk JD, Nau J, Reichel E, Singer M, Barak A, Binder S, Jackson TL: Epimacular brachytherapy for neovascular age-related macular degeration. A randomized, control trial (CABERNET). Ophthalmology 2013;120:317–327.
12 Bianciotto C, Shields CL, Pirondini C, Mashayekhi A, Furuta M, Shields JA: Proliferative radiation retinopathy after plaque radiotherapy for uveal melanoma. Ophthalmology 2010;117:1005–1012.
13 Shields CL, Naseripour M, Cater J, Shields JA, Demirci H, Youseff A, Freire J: Plaque radiotherapy for large posterior uveal melanoma (>8 mm thick) in 354 consecutive patients. Ophthalmology 2002;109: 1838–1849.
14 Groenewald C, Konstantinidis L, Damato B: Effects of radiotherapy on uveal melanoma and adjacent tissues. Eye (Lond) 2013;27:163–171.
15 Dunavoelgyi R, Dieckmann K, Gleiss A, Sacu S, Kircher K, Georgopoulos M, Georg D, Zehetmayer M, Poetter R: Radiogenic side effects after hypofractionated stereotactic photon radiotherapy of choroidal melanoma in 212 patients treated between 1997 and 2007. Int J Radiat Oncol Biol Phys 2012;83:121–128.
16 Guyer DR, Mukai S, Egan KM, Seddon JM, Walsh SM, Gragoudas ES: Radiation maculopathy after proton beam irradiation for choroidal melanoma. Ophthalmology 1992;99:1278–1285.
17 Marcocci C, Bartalena L, Rocchi R, Marino M, Menconi F, Morabito E, Mazzi B, Mazzeo S, Sartini MS, Nardi M, Cartei F, Cionini L, Pinchera A: Long-term safety of orbital radiotherapy for Graves' ophthalmopathy. J Clin Endocrinol Metab 2003;88:3561–3566.
18 Wakelkamp IM, Tan H, Saeed P, Schlingemann RO, Verbraak FD, Blank LECM, Prummel MF, Wiersinga WM: Orbital irradiation for Graves' ophthalmopathy. Is it safe? A long-term follow-up study. Ophthalmology 2004;111:1557–1562.
19 Giuliari GP, Sadaka A, Hinkle DM, Simpson ER: Current treatment for radiation retinopathy. Acta Oncol 2011;50:6–13.
20 Ahuja Y, Kapoor KG, Thompson RM, Furutani KM, Shultz RW, Stafford SL, Dev S, Abu-Yaghi NE, Reynolds D, Pulido JS: The effects of intraocular silicone oil placement prior to iodine 125 brachytherapy for uveal melanoma: a clinical case series. Eye 2012;26: 1487–1489.
21 Singh AD, Pabon S, Aronow ME: Management of radiation maculopathy. Ophthalmic Res 2012;48: 26–31.
22 Mayo C, Martel MK, Marks LB, Flickinger J, Nam J, Kirkpatrick J: Radiation dose-volume effects of optic nerves and chiasm. Int J Radiat Oncol Biol Phys 2010;76:S28–S35.
23 Danesh-Meyer HV: Radiation-induced optic neuropathy. J Clin Neurosci 2008;15:95–100.
24 Jiang GL, Tucker SL, Gutenberg R, Peters LJ, Morrison WH, Garden AS, Ha CS, Ang KK: Radiation-induced injury to the optic pathway. Radiother Oncol 1994;30:17–25.
25 Stafford SL, Pollock BE, Leavitt JA, Foote RL, Brown PD, Link MJ, Gorman DA, Schomberg PJ: A study on radiation tolerance of the optic nerves and chiasm after stereotactic radiosurgery. Int J Radiat Biol Phys 2003;55:1177–1181.
26 Leber KA, Berglöff J, Pendl G: Dose-response tolerance of the visual pathways and cranial nerves of the cavernous sinus to stereotactic radiosurgery. J Neurosurg 1998;88:43–50.
27 Puusaari I, Heikkonen J, Kivelä T: Effect of radiation dose on ocular complications after iodine brachytherapy for large uveal melanoma: empirical data and simulation of collimating plaques. Invest Ophthalmol Vis Sci 2004;45:3425–3434.
28 Puusaari I, Heikkonen J, Kivelä T: Ocular complications after iodine brachytherapy for large uveal melanomas. Ophthalmology 2004;111:1768–1777.
29 Sánchez-Orgaz M, Grabowska A, Roya-Oreja A, Asecio-Durán M, Romero-Mártin R, Arbizu-Duralde A: Optic neuropathy following orbital irradiation for Graves' ophthalmopathy: a case report and literature review. Orbit 2012;31:30–33.
30 Kim IK, Lane A-M, Egan KM, Munzenrider J, Gragoudas ES: Natural history of radiation papillopathy after proton beam irradiatioin of parapapillary melanoma. Ophthalmology 2010;117:1617–1622.
31 Krama H, Heydarian M, Beiki-Ardakani A, Weisbrod D, Xu W, Simpson RE, Sahqal A: A comparison between 125-iodine brachytherapy and stereotactic radiotherapy in the management of juxtapapillary choroidal melanoma. Br J Ophthalmol 2013;97:327–332.
32 Parsons JT, Bova FJ, Fitzgerald CR, Mendenhall WM, Million RR: Radiation optic neuropathy after mega voltage external-beam irradiation: analysis of time-dose factors. Int J Radiat Oncol Biol Phys 1994; 31:1041–1042.
33 Bhandare N, Monroe AT, Morris CG, Bhatti MT, Mendenhall WM: Does altered fractionation influence the risk of radiation-induced optic neuropathy? Int J Radiat Oncol Biol Phys 2005;62:1070–1077.
34 Miller NR: Radiation-induced optic neuropathy: still no treatment. Clin Exp Ophthalmol 2004;32:233–235.

35 Correa Z, Augsburger JJ, Freire J, Eagle RC Jr: Early-onset scleral necrosis after iodine 125 plaque radiotherapy for ciliochoroidal melanoma. Arch Ophthalmol 1999;117:259–261.
36 Chaudry IA, Liu M, Shamsi FA, Arat YO, Shetlar DJ, Boniuk M: Corneoscleral necrosis after episcleral Au-198 brachytherapy of uveal melanoma. Retina 2009;29:73–79.
37 Radin PR, Lumbroso-Le Rouic L, Levy-Gabriel C, Dendale R, Sastre X, Desjardins L: Scleral necrosis after radiation therapy for uveal melanomas: report of 23 cases. Graefes Arch Clin Exp Ophthalmol 2008;246:1731–1736.
38 Barman M, Finger PT, Milman T: Scleral patch graft in the management of uveal and ocular surface tumors. Ophthalmology 2012;119:2631–2636.
39 Gündüz K, Shields CL, Shields JA, Cater J, Freire JE, Brady LW: Plaque radiotherapy of uveal melanoma with predominantly ciliary body involvement. Arch Ophthalmol 1999;117:170–177.
40 Gündüz K, Shields CL, Shields JA, Cater J, Freire JE, Brady LW: Plaque radiotherapy for management of ciliary body and choroidal melanoma with extraocular extension. Am J Ophthalmol 2000;130:97–102.
41 Kaiserman N, Kaiserman I, Hendler K, Frenkel S, Pe'er J: Rutehenium-106 brachytherapy for thick posterior uveal melanoma. Br J Ophthalmol 2009;93:1167–1171.
42 Bergman L, Nilsson B, Lundell G, Lundell M, Seregard S: Ruthenium brachytherapy for uveal melanoma, 1979–2003. Survival and functional outcome in the Swedish population. Ophthalmology 2005;112:834–840.

David E. Pelayes, MD
Full Professor, Ophthalmology, Maimonides University and
Associate Professor, Ophthalmology, Buenos Aires University
Buenos Aires (Argentina)
E-Mail davidpelayes@gmail.com

Subject Index